WHAT IS, AS IT IS

SATSANGS WITH PRABHUJI

WHAT IS, AS IT IS

SATSANGS WITH *Prabhuji*

WHAT IS, AS IT IS
SATSANGS WITH PRABHUJI

Tenth Edition
Printed in the United States of America

Published by Prabhuji Mission
Website: prabhuji.net

Prabhuji Ashram
PO Box 900
Cairo, NY, 12413
USA

Painting on the cover by Prabhuji:
"Meeting"
Acrylic on canvas, New York
Canvas Size: 48" x 48"

Library of Congress Control Number: 2015933180
ISBN-13: 978-0-9815264-4-7

Table of Contents

Preface 9
Introduction 13
A Door to the Infinite 17
Seek your Posture in Life 25
Asana - the Vital Yogic Posture 35
Discover the Magic of Repetition 43
Karma Yoga - the Art of Action 53
Action and Reaction in Karma Yoga 61
Communion 67
Repression and Sublimation 75
Desire 83
Jump into the Real Dimension 91
Desire Hides Reality from us 97
Meditation - the Path to Freedom 105
Observing the Internal Conflict 111
Self-Investigation 119
Seeking the Seeker 123
What is, as it is 131

Appendix

Glossary of Sanskrit Terms 139
Index of Verses 153
Biography 159
About the Prabhuji Mission 169
About the Prabhuji Ashram 171
The path of Transcendental Consciousness 173
Important clarification 175

With deep gratitude and respect, this book is dedicated to my beloved masters.

Preface

The story of my life is nothing more than a long journey, from what I believed myself to be to what I truly am. It is a tale of transcending the personal and the universal, the partial and the total, the illusory and the real, the apparent and the true. My life is a flight beyond the temporal and the eternal, darkness and light, the human and the divine. This story is not public but profoundly private and intimate.

Only what begins, ends; only what starts, finishes. One who lives in the present is neither born nor dies, because what lacks a beginning never ends.

I am the disciple of a seer, an enlightened being, somebody who is nobody. I was initiated in my spiritual childhood by the moonlight. A seagull who loved flying more than anything else in life inspired me. In love with the impossible, I crossed the universe obsessed with a star. I have walked infinite paths, following the footsteps of those who saw.

Like the ocean that longs for water, I sought my home within my own house.

I am a simple intermediary who shares his experience with others. I am not a guide, teacher, instructor, educator, psychologist, enlightener, pedagogue, evangelist, rabbi, *posek halacha*, healer, therapist, satsangist, psychic, leader, medium, savior, or guru, but only a traveler whom you can ask for directions. I will gladly show you a place where everything calms upon arrival, a place beyond the sun and the stars, beyond your desires and longings, beyond time and space, beyond concepts and conclusions, beyond everything that you believe you are or imagine that you will be.

I am just a whim and maybe a joke from the sky and the only mistake of my beloved spiritual master.

Aware of the abyss that separates revelation and our works, we live in a frustrated attempt to faithfully express the mystery of the spirit.

I paint sighs, hopes, silences, aspirations, and melancholies… inner landscapes and sunsets of the soul.

I am a painter of the indescribable, inexpressible, and indefinable of our depths… and maybe I just write colors and paint words.

Since childhood, little windows of paper captivated my attention; through them, I visited places, met people, and made friends. Those tiny *maṇḍalas* were my true elementary school, high school, and college. Like skilled teachers, these *yantras* have guided me through contemplation, attention, concentration, observation, and meditation.

Like a physician studies the human body, or a lawyer studies laws, I have dedicated my entire life to study myself. I can say with certainty that I know what resides and lives in this heart.

It is not my intention to convince anyone of anything. I neither offer a theology or philosophy, nor do I preach or teach, I simply think out loud. The echo of these words may lead you to the infinite space of peace, silence, love, existence, consciousness, and absolute bliss.

Do not waste your precious time searching for me, but search for yourself. You do not need me or anyone else, because the only thing that really matters is you. What you yearn for lies within you, as what you are, here and now.

I am not a merchant of recycled information nor do I intend to trade with my spiritual state. I do not teach beliefs or philosophies but speak only about what I see and share solely what I know.

Avoid fame, for true glory is not based on public opinion but on what you really are. What matters is not what others think of you, but your own appreciation of who you are.

Choose bliss over success, life over reputation, and wisdom over information. If you succeed, you will know not only admiration but also true envy. However, jealousy is a tribute that mediocrity pays to talent: it is merely acceptance and an open declaration of inferiority.

I advise you to fly freely and never be afraid of making mistakes. Learn the art of transforming your errors into lessons. Never blame others for your faults: remember that taking complete responsibility for your life is a sign of maturity. When you fly, you learn that what matters is not touching the sky but the courage to spread your wings. The higher you rise, the smaller and less significant the world looks. As you walk, sooner or later you will understand that every search begins and ends in you.

Your unconditional well-wisher,
Prabhuji

Introduction

Excerpt from a satsang given by Prabhuji on April 18, 2010

These meetings aren't lessons or lectures; they can only be called *satsaṅgs,* or "meetings with the Truth." *Satsaṅga* is a Sanskrit word composed of two terms: *sat* or *satya*, "Truth," and *saṅga*. *Saṅga* is a word that we find in so many different places: *sādhu-saṅga*, the *saṅga* of the disciples of Lord Buddha. *Saṅga* is "together," "in community," "gathered."

A lesson or conference is a meeting on a verbal or mental level, an encounter on the level of words, of the intellect. It's the meeting between a teacher and students in which study takes place. From a meeting of minds, only knowledge can ensue, but wisdom can never blossom as it can only arise from *saṅga*.

The meeting between students and their teacher provides a place for communication; they may be close, but never together. *Saṅga* can only happen in communion, not in communication. Communion is a meeting between souls at the level of the spirit, of the heart, of a presence.

Truth is born in unity. That's why what matters in this kind of event is not the information, but the fact of being together. More important than words and phrases is to what they refer. Everything lies in this togetherness.

It's remarkable that we can be very near physically, yet so far. Like those couples we may meet at weddings who have been married for many years. They sit at the same table, however, they appear aloof toward one another; they might live in the same house and sleep in the same bed, yet the abysmal distance that separates them can't be measured in kilometers, meters or miles. On the other hand, you may happen to know people who, for one reason or another, have been separated from loved ones and in spite of being so far away physically, one may notice that their hearts are in another place, with the other person.

Similarly, the hearts of the master and disciple live together, truly together, and that's what happens in a satsang: a "being together," unity, a kind of yoga. The *Bhagavad-gītā* (chapter 4, verse 34) states:

tad viddhi praṇipātena
paripraśnena sevayā
upadekṣyanti te jñānaṁ
jñāninas tattva-darśinaḥ

If you wish to find the Truth, approach a spiritual master, inquire submissively, and with humility, offer service. One who has seen the Truth can transmit it to you, can show it to you.

The disciple must inquire, but that does not mean to have many questions, rather to *be* a question; because to be a question is to put aside all that you know. It's to renounce every idea or conclusion and stand naked in front of someone who is *tattva-darśin*, who has seen the Truth.

The more I strip myself of what I believe I know—of my points of view, my preconceived ideas—the more I get rid of my isolation and come closer. The moment I don't know, I don't simply ask; rather I become a question. I have no answers because any answer will come from the past, from the information that I've acquired in my life, from knowledge, from the known. These are not *my* answers.

The disciple is someone who has understood the following:

> I don't have my own answers! Sure, I can answer: I know about Egyptian civilization, Napoleon, arithmetic, geography, I know where Brazil and Spain are, but these answers are not *mine*. They are what I have acquired through my contact with society: teachers from school, university, parents, friends, etc. I've made and accumulated images, and now I have a large collection of them. I can answer any question by presenting an image, but this knowledge that I've acquired from the external world is not mine!

As a disciple, I have no answers, I am just a question. I'm humble enough to say, "I don't know," and that is to come closer: *saṅga*, joined, together.

In order to be *really* together, we need to establish ourselves as disciples: renouncing our answers, our points of view, our ideas, concepts, and conclusions... then what difference can exist between you and me, between her and another person?

We are together and in that togetherness, satsang is born and Truth blossoms. We *are* Truth.

A Door to the Infinite

July 13, 2010

There is confusion among Westerners regarding hatha yoga, asanas, and yoga in general. There are people who attend classes on yogic philosophy, and when asked what yoga is, they say, "Well, yoga is a Hindu philosophy," and they describe students listening to a teacher. Some people practice meditation in some of the several workshops or institutions that teach it, and when asked what yoga is, they say that yoga is meditation and they describe people with closed eyes. And, of course, there are those who practice hatha yoga in different studios or centers. They go with their mats and are typically quite preoccupied with everything related to health. Then, when you ask them what yoga is, they say that yoga is a very healthy method to stay in shape. Each person is trying to define yoga, and everyone is right, but yoga isn't just that.

There are those who compare yoga to a tree in which the roots are *yama*, the trunk is *niyama*, and the sap is hatha yoga, which gives vitality to the whole body. The leaves may be compared to *prāṇāyāma*, and the bark to *pratyāhāra*, or "the internalization of the senses," which holds the tree together in a certain shape and doesn't allow it to fall apart. *Dhāraṇā* would be the branches, and *dhyāna*, the fruit, because meditation is the fruit of yoga; it still has a purpose, like the fruit that provides nutrition. Lastly, *samādhi*, or "enlightenment," is the flower that has no purpose; it is pure beauty, color, fragrance.

So, to take one part of yoga and try to define it through that aspect—removing it from the context of the entire tree—will always be a grave error. It's true that yoga is also physical, just like the tree is the root, the trunk, and the leaves. Although if we look at hatha yoga within its context, we will see that the physical aspect is like a passage, or a gate: it's there to reach something further.

Yoga is about knowing and studying in order to be able to observe and then to transcend. For example, raja yoga is to know the mind in order to transcend it. Likewise, the asana is getting to know the body, to study it, and to pass through it, like through a door.

In his *Yoga Sūtra* (2.46-48), Patañjali Maharishi tells us:

sthira-sukham āsanam

Asanas should be stable and comfortable.

prayatna-śaithilyānanta-samāpattibhyām

The asana is achieved by eliminating tension and meditating.

tato dvandvānabhighātaḥ

> In achieving the asana, one also attains immunity from the pairs of opposites.

In these sutras we find great secrets. What is hatha yoga? *Sthira-sukham āsanam* means that the asana is firm, comfortable, and stable: that is a posture. Why is it so important that it be firm and comfortable?

We must understand that the *Sanātana-dharma* religion suggests an educational process that is very different from what we're used to. In our life, we are accustomed to the fact that studying is memorizing. The more we remember, the more we know and the more tests we are able to pass: we need to remember who the Egyptians are, and Napoleon, and how the Spartans fought the battle of Thermopylae, remember and remember!

On the contrary, religion is a process of forgetting. The more you forget, the closer you are to your home, to the place you never left. Thus, in hatha yoga we try to forget the body. Notice that we remember the body when we have problems: a headache comes to remind us that we have a head; arthritis, our bones; a torn muscle, our muscular system. In other words, what the pain, ache, and discomfort do is they remind us of our body. Likewise, an asana—being firm, stable, and comfortable—leads us to a state of forgetfulness of the body.

Forgetting the body isn't simple; it's to forget a concept that we live by: the corporeal concept of life. Hatha yoga leads us to forget our form: we forget ourselves as a limitation in space and in time, as *someone*; we forget ourselves as an objectified phenomenon. This happens when we are comfortable.

The process of hatha yoga, through asanas, leads us to adjust to the body. We're living with the body, but uncomfortably. However, these discomforts are overcome after forgetting the body; we can go on to forget many other things: for example, the incredible human invention that is the ego, or the "I." Imagine what we would have done without ego, without this concept, without the I-idea! How would we communicate? How would it be possible to relate to one another? It would be completely impossible! Nevertheless, this is a fantastic creation.

But to live all our life concerned with the "I"—I want, I don't want, I like, I don't like, and I'm the only important one—is a sickness called *egoism*, which is an obsession with the "I." We can't forget it: it's like a headache that constantly reminds us of the head. Egoism continuously reminds us of this "I," and it neither lets us forget it nor act freely. In a more advanced level of yoga, you come to *forget* yourself.

But the body is a door; it's the beginning. A forgotten body is like an open door: you pass through it without feeling any obstacle. If you feel the door, then it must be closed: you feel it in front of your face and you can't pass. In this way, when the body is comfortable and forgotten, you can pass through without feeling it. When you forget the mind, it's the door to the infinite, to eternity.

Patañjali says in sutra 47:

prayatna-śaithilyānanta-samāpattibhyām

> The asana is achieved by eliminating tension and meditating.

Meditating: The asana is a state of meditation.

And sutra 48:

tato dvandvānabhighāta

> In achieving the asana, one also attains immunity from the pairs of opposites.

The pairs of opposites are transcended when we obtain mastery of the asana. This sounds very strange to many people: how is it possible to transcend the pairs of opposites through a posture of the physical body?

The pairs of opposites are the mind. The mind moves constantly like a little bee seeking happiness from one flower to the next.

> Maybe I'll be happy with this chocolate.
> Maybe I'll be happy with this cigarette.
> No! I'll be happier with this beer.
> Better yet, with this music... with this television... with this new car...
> I'll get married and be happy... or when I have children...

The mind constantly rambles in the pairs of opposites, in the duality of attraction and rejection, attachment and aversion. We are internally broken, living fractured and in conflict: something can be so pleasant and comfortable... but it's bad; and something can be so difficult and inconvenient... but it's good. We understand the conflict, the internal struggle, the pairs of opposites, and that constant mental movement. But how can we transcend it through a physical posture?

In order to grasp this, we must understand what the sages of antiquity revealed long ago: the mind and body aren't two different phenomena, but simply two aspects of the same one. They are like two ends of the same rope. The body is nothing more than the exteriorization of the mind. The senses are the mind externalizing itself.

When we see, it's the mind that sees, not the eyes. When we touch, it's the mind that touches; when we smell something, it's the mind that smells. Through the body, it's the mind that moves in the world of names and forms, in the world of the relative. Because the mind and the body are the same thing, our mental state is reflected in our physical postures. We can tell if others are annoyed, happy, content, sad, or tired by the many physical postures, expressions, or gestures because the mind and the body are so interrelated, they are one and the same.

The asana is static. When the asana occurs and the body stops all movement, then something happens on the mental level, or rather, something ceases on the mental level. Movement begins to diminish. You've taken over the mind but from the side nearest to you: the body. From the body, you can affect the mind, you can influence the mind with the asana, the art of stopping.

You shouldn't repress: Patañjali tells us that the asana should be comfortable, not forced, not against the body, rather with the body: you should come to the mastery of knowing how to stop. And when you have managed to become motionless—without moving physically and comfortable—the moment arrives in which the mind desists; the conflict between the pairs of opposites ceases. And when the division, the internal fracture, the movement, the internal action stops... there is no mind! Because the mind is movement, the intrinsic reality of the mind is movement.

And from here comes the moment of forgetting: first the body is forgotten in order to finally forget the mind. The mind is forgotten, but *you* don't forget it, because when the mind stops, you are forgetting yourself, in order to emerge in remembrance. You're forgetting what you believe yourself to be, what you think you are, what you've been convinced that you are, what you've been told you are, what you recall yourself to be, in order to emerge from that forgetting, to emerge in remembrance, where existence is remembered, and that's the remembrance of what you truly are.

The body is the first door toward deeper, more internal levels. The mind is the last door: when you cross that door you are no one, but you are. You are, but you *are* not someone. Nothing changes, but nothing will be the same.

Seek your Posture in Life

July 17, 2010

Hatha yoga is perhaps the most ancient psycho-physiological system known to humanity; it begins with the practice of asanas, or "postures." The asana is the third limb of Patañjali Maharishi's *aṣṭāṅga-yoga* system. To better understand what is an asana, it's important to refer to Patañjali's *Yoga Sūtra*.

The *Yoga Sūtra* is divided into four chapters called *pādas*, or "feet." Just like a table needs four legs in order to stand, so the *Yoga Sūtra* is supported by four *pādas*. These four chapters are written in sutras, which are like capsules that contain the maximum wisdom within the minimum amount of words.

In the *sādhana-pāda* (chapter 2), sutra 46, Patañjali explains what an asana is:

sthira-sukham āsanam

That is a posture: *sthira-sukham āsanam*, it is steady and comfortable; in other words, when you feel steady and comfortable, you are in an asana, although not every position can be called an asana.

Sutra 47 says:

prayatna-śaithilyānanta-samāpattibhyām

> The asana is achieved by eliminating tension and meditating on the infinite.

This gives us a guide, a direction, on how to reach the asana, how to find it and be situated in it.

And sutra 48 says:

tato dvandvānabhighātaḥ

> In accomplishing the asana [in attaining mastery over the asana], one also attains immunity from the pairs of opposites.

We are going to examine these three sutras deeper in order to better understand what an asana is. Sutra 46 says:

sthira-sukham āsanam

> The asana is stable and comfortable.

Most of us practice hatha yoga and know what an asana is: it is to remain in a specific posture for a certain period of time, steady, stable, comfortable, in watchfulness, and in a meditative state.

There are those who try to divide postures into physical and meditative, but actually, every posture is as meditative as it is physical. What happens is that before we have attained mastery over the posture, we think it's physical because we are still struggling and making efforts to reach it. So we relate to it as something physical. However, when some mastery has been achieved, we refer to it as a meditative posture.

To delve into the subject of the yogic posture, it will be essential to understand that the Vedic sages of antiquity—and yoga in general—clearly do not consider the physical body as disconnected from the mind. The psychic and physical planes are not separate. Much to the contrary, they are different aspects of the same phenomenon. The mind is the body; the body is the mind. The body is an externalization of the mind. It is the mind moving on the physical plane.

According to *Sanātana-dharma*—from which yoga originates—human beings are not something as simple as physical bodies with souls inside. Rather, they comprise many facets, levels, and aspects: physical, mental, emotional, energetic… Therefore, when Patañjali speaks to us about a posture, clearly, he isn't referring *solely* to a physical position; when he says that the asana is steady and comfortable, he's referring to the body, as well as all that the human being encompasses.

After this introduction, we can begin to examine the steadiness and comfort of the asana.

According to yoga, disease is one of the great obstacles on the retroprogressive process. Not only because disease prevents us from being able to study or have association with our spiritual master, there's much more to it: pain, discomfort, and uneasiness remind us of the body. When we have a migraine, we remember the head; indigestion reminds us of the stomach; a sprain reminds us of the muscle. Of course, this causes us great discomfort on the mental level because the body and the mind are related.

The posture must, therefore, be comfortable and stable. When you feel comfortable, a process of forgetting the body occurs. When there is no indigestion, you don't remember your stomach; when there is no sprain and the muscles are comfortable, you don't feel them, you forget them; you forget your head when there is no migraine and you see it as a great orifice in the universe from which you observe everything that happens.

When placing yourself in the comfortable asana, you forget your anatomy; a forgetfulness of your physical aspect occurs, which includes much more than the body. It is the forgetting of an attitude toward life, a concept: your bodily attitude toward life.

What do we forget? Not only our limitation of space and time—our form—but also the concept that I am the body, that I was born on the day that the body appeared, that I love all those who, in one way or another, are related to this body: my children, my wife, my nieces and nephews, my grandchildren, my compatriots, because they are an expansion of my body. To forget is to cease searching for happiness and bliss through the body and the senses, to stop giving it champagne or smoke; because if I desire happiness and I am the body, then the way to be happy is by offering the body pleasure and enjoying it. However, we continue to be just as miserable because we are not *only* the body. It is one of our aspects, but it isn't everything.

To be situated in the asana is to forget the very limited concept we have of ourselves and of life; it's to forget the body and the worship of the geographical place from where it came into this world: I am Chilean, Chile is the most glorious country! I am British, England is the most powerful country! I am Russian, Russia is the motherland!

If we forget ourselves on the physical level, sooner or later we will forget ourselves on the mental level because body and mind are two aspects of the same phenomenon, the same reality. Through the body, we can learn what is happening in a person on the mental level: sadness, happiness, enjoyment, jealousy, anger. All this is reflected on our faces and in our physical postures.

All that happens in the mind is expressed through the body. Even lie detectors can identify electric reactions in the body because what is happening in the mind is expressed in the brain, and what is happening in the brain is expressed in the body. The mind and the body are like two ends of the same cord. In this way, in the asana, you forget the body and at the mental level, forgetfulness of the mind occurs.

Why is this forgetting so important? We have been taught to remember, to memorize. Since grade school, to learn has meant to remember for a test: if we remember what they ask us, we pass and succeed; if we don't remember, we are in trouble. To remember is to know, to remember is to progress.

On the path of religion, in the spiritual field, it is exactly the opposite: it is a process of forgetting, for the simple reason that the ego is memory and remembrance. Therefore, if the path of religion is to transcend the ego, transcending ourselves will be to forget.

We are memory, we are the recollection of all opinions or ideas and of all that has been said about us. From the first moment that they told us our name: "You are Joseph, you are John, you are Rose, you are Miriam, that is who you are..." We remembered it.

Afterwards, we continued remembering opinions: you are pretty, you are ugly, you are smart, you are an unbearable person, you are a teacher, a doctor, etc. However, of this entire aggregate of opinions, not one is your own, not one is your own discovery: they are a collection of external opinions concerning what you are, whose authority is another person; but you are not the authority of any of them.

When we're asked who or what we are, we whip out the list: I am Chilean, I am Russian, I am Argentinean, I am from here, I am from there, I am John, I am Michael, I am Mary; and we go on... This has led us to so many inferiority complexes! It is all on the list: I am a doctor, a teacher, a bank teller, etc. This pile of ideas is the ego. Now, to transcend this I-idea is exactly to forget, because the mind is remembering. One who is capable of forgetting the body can achieve the process of this forgetfulness gradually occurring at every level.

And how is this attained? Patañjali tells us in sutra 47:

prayatna-śaithilyānanta-samāpattibhyām

> The asana, or "posture," is reached by eliminating tension and meditating on the infinite.

This is what we have been accustomed to in life: *How* do we achieve? *How* do we do? *How* do we get? We must strive for all that we desire, aspire to, and want because we are acting from a place of lacking, of absence. We go through life with the deep impression that we're missing something, and we believe that by possessing—and to possess one must strive—we will succeed in filling this void. You do not realize that *you* are what is missing. The one who is not present here and now is *you*.

The ego is an immense pit into which we are constantly throwing things: objects, money, fame, honor, people... This pit never closes, instead it keeps on growing. We've been taught to strive, to do. The ego is the great actor that does in order to obtain, to achieve.

That inheres in society, in this world. However, in the sphere of religion, in the spiritual realm, if you want to obtain spiritual benefits—like meditation, enlightenment, God, the soul—then relaxation is required. These benefits need an opportunity in order to emerge; in other words, you need to eliminate tension. Tension is a kind of obstacle for the occurrence of *yourself*, for consciousness to happen, for heaven to caress you. Tension and anxiety are obstacles: every spiritual benefit comes when you relax.

You can only attain what you are when you do not try to obtain it because in trying to reach it, there is tension, there is anxiety. To eliminate tension is to transcend the ego, because the ego is tension and anxiety. Thus, this elimination of tension is the way to reach the asana, your posture; and when the posture occurs, meditation will occur.

The posture is much more than a physical pose; we also take a posture toward a situation or a person, toward life. It's not just a physical meaning, it's also an attitude. If you look around and see the world and the people going from here to there—from one job to another, from one house to another, from one profession to another—you'll see that everyone is seeking *the posture* because no one is stable.

We are susceptible to being moved by illusion, desires, or temptations, and we are always seeking something more. Because we feel so uncomfortable! We seek the posture. To find the posture is to find ourselves because when we find the place, we find the one who is situated in that place. To find the posture is to situate ourselves, and that is what we are all seeking: to become situated in *our place.*

Where is the stable and comfortable place? In sutra 48, Patañjali says:

tato dvandvānabhighātaḥ

> In accomplishing the asana, one also attains immunity from the pairs of opposites.

The mind doesn't move, rather it *is* movement; the mind is activity. This is why Patañjali Maharishi says, at the beginning of the *Yoga Sūtra*: *yogaś citta-vṛtti-nirodhaḥ*, which means that yoga is a state in which the mind is quiet and there is no mental movement of the *vṛttis*. Therefore, when we attain mastery over the asana and situate ourselves in it, the body manages to become still and similarly the mind becomes still: there is no mental movement and there are no more mental waves.

Since the mind is movement and activity, upon stopping… it no longer exists! A quiet mind is a mind that isn't there because the mind is like a dance: when we cease to move, there is no dance. Dance is the movement itself. If we are dancing, there is a dance; but if we stop, there is no dance... Likewise, the mind is the movement of the *vṛttis*, or thoughts, but when the mind attains that steady state and ceases to move, there is no mind.

You are the mind, so in that stillness of the asana, you're absent; you're not someone, but you are. That is to say, you're there as a presence but your concepts, ideas, and opinions dissipate. It is said that the world disappears when the ego vanishes, but what disappears is *your* world: your way of seeing and interpreting it. You cease to be there as a separate entity, disconnected from the universe. It is the disappearance of what you think you are, of what you believe yourself to be, of that accumulation of opinions that you have been told you are. Rather, you are present as what you really are, your authenticity, and your reality.

Patañjali says: *sthira-sukham āsanam*, "the asana must be firm and comfortable." Everyone is going around seeking his or her posture in life. To find it is to find yourself. It's no coincidence that in Genesis, chapter 3, verse 9, the omniscient, all-knowing God asks Adam a question. He asks, *"Ayeka?"* "Where art thou?" For many years, I asked myself how it could be that God, who is omniscient, did not know where Adam was. Finally, I reached the conclusion that rather than a question, it's advice: "Where art thou?" Search for where you are among all the things that belong to you: my house, my country, my family, my body, my foot, my hand, my head, my heart, my brain, my mind, my spirit, my soul; but where is that which you can call the "I"? If you find out where you are, if you place yourself... you discover yourself.

The seat of the guru is special. The disciples sit on the floor and the guru is seated on a big chair that is called a *vyāsāsan*, or "the asana of Vyāsa." This is because it is reserved for someone who has found his or her asana, the original asana.

If you find the posture here, where *you* are—not where your body, your mind, or your thoughts are—if you put yourself firmly in the here, nothing can move you, not illusion, desires, nor fantasies, so steady and so comfortable that nothing in the universe can entice you.

It is said that such beings, wherever they go—even if they talk and move throughout all the universes, like Nārada, never move from the now. Someone who is unmoved by memories, nostalgia, imagination, or future ambitions, is always situated in the now, *only* in the now, moving in the eternal now, in the eternal moment… not moving in or from the past, rather situated in the now, in the here.

To seek the asana is to seek yourself. "Where am I?" is like asking yourself, "Who am I?" The discovery is a revelation that in the dual world of relativity, we seek pleasure, enjoyment, and happiness; and when they speak to us about enlightenment—of finding ourselves or of finding our posture—we may think they're speaking of a great pleasure or happiness. But those who know would say otherwise: the realization of your authentic nature brings you to the comfort of being in the place where you belong, of being what you are. It's that type of comfort from which nothing can tempt you because there can be no greater pleasure.

Comfort is your place; your place is transcendental comfort.

Asana - the Vital Yogic Posture

July 25, 2010

To understand what an asana is, it is best to turn to the *Yoga Sūtra* of Patañjali Maharishi; no one else has accomplished such a compilation about yoga. In his chapter 2, sutra 46, he speaks to us about *sādhana*:

sthira-sukham āsanam

An asana is stable and comfortable.

We must understand that yoga does not view the mind as something separate from the body. In other words, hatha yoga isn't considered to be simply a physical or bodily discipline, but one directed toward every aspect of the human being: the physical and mental aspect, as well as the emotional and energetic.

Therefore, when Patañjali refers to the asana, he means much more than just a physical posture. We can't just take it as a gymnastic practice or physical training, for he isn't just referring to the placement of our body; rather to the *posture.*

What is your posture in life?

Over so many years and reincarnations, it seems that everyone changes postures, from bachelor to spouse, from spouse to parent. We are constantly seeking: to be millionaires, famous, doctors, lawyers, soldiers, Americans, Italians, etc. That is to say, we look around and see that practically everyone is seeking to change their position, as if we all walk about in search of our position.

Patañjali says that we can recognize our asana, or "posture": after this long search, you will know when you have reached the posture because it will be firm, stable, and comfortable, *sthira-sukham āsanam.* Presently, if you examine yourself, you will see that your own posture in the universe is not steady; it is inconsistent because you do not feel comfortable.

One of the meanings of the word *guru* is "heavy," implying that nothing can move him or her. Desires move us, ambitions move us, the search for pleasure and enjoyment moves us. We aren't steady.

It's quite interesting that the word *asana* specifically refers to the seated posture. It isn't a standing posture, which has *rajas* in it, as there is an effort to remain standing; neither does it refer to a reclining posture, because that would be tamasic. The asana is neither one extreme nor the other. It is to be seated, but steady, motionless, so that nothing can move you from your posture in life. But not out of repression, not because it should be this way, not out of a struggle against the body or against yourself; rather, the asana should be steady, stable, and comfortable.

Once at ease, there is no need to move. Meaning, if we move in life—from being single to married, from being married to a parent, from parent to doctor or professor, and from there, to become a millionaire or famous—it's because we are not comfortable: we haven't found the posture that would be stable and comfortable.

Mind and body are the same thing: the posture is as physical as it is mental, emotional, or energetic; it's about finding your posture in life. When the physical posture is firm and comfortable, we forget our physical aspect, we forget the body.

Any discomfort or disease reminds you of the body: a headache reminds you of the head, indigestion reminds you of the stomach, a sprain reminds you of a muscle, etc. A painful organ reminds you of itself because something is not functioning well. Thus, discomfort reminds you of the body; but when there is comfort, you forget the body.

In material life, if we want to obtain something, we must remember; for example, when we study in school we understand that to pass the grade, we must remember, so we will progress. But in religion, it is exactly the opposite: it's the path of forgetting for the simple reason that *we are* memorization, *we are* memory.

The ego is memory, as it's everything that its remember about itself; you are your name, your nationality, your family, and many behavioral patterns that you've acquired. Therefore, the process of transcending the ego is the process of forgetting. Religious life is a forgetting of the body and of all the different aspects: physical, energetic, mental, etc.

Hence, the body would be the first door leading to that state, to that asana in which I'm steady and relaxed, in such a way that the body is forgotten. Later, the mind is forgotten, because just as when the body is firm and comfortable and so forgotten, we also forget the mind. A steady, comfortable mind is simply forgotten… and forgetting what you believe yourself to be is realizing what you really are.

One who seeks results always wants the "how," the technique, and asks: "How do we reach this steadiness and comfort in the asana?" In sutra 47, Patañjali tells us:

prayatna-śaithilyānanta-samāpattibhyām

> The asana is achieved by eliminating tension and meditating.

That is to say, to arrive at the posture, one must eliminate tension. This is something so different from what we have been used to in life! We are accustomed to struggle to obtain things; we need to make efforts and great sacrifices, which involve tension: the tension of ambition and of desire. If you want to obtain money or fame, you must strive and live in tension.

In spiritual life, however, benefits don't come through effort, but through the elimination of tension. Your posture in life won't be found by trying to be this or that. If you want to find your position in life, you can't be moving from here to there, seeking and striving.

In order to reach this steadiness and comfort, all you need to do is eliminate tension and forget the body. By forgetting the "I," you're relieved of the horrible disease of egoism, which consists in a constant remembrance. Just as you remember the head because of your migraine, the stomach because of your indigestion, the muscle because of your sprain; due to your egoism, you can't stop remembering the "I": I want this, I want that, I don't want this, I like this, I like that. The "I" is the most important thing: we live our entire lives defending that "I," inflating it, taking care of it, and protecting it. There is hunger in Africa and India, but what matters is that *I* eat. There is sadness, but most importantly, *I* am sad. There is poverty, but *I* should not be poor. People suffer, but the horror is if *I* suffer. If others are suffering, it's not *my* problem!

The "I" continually reminds us—like a toothache—indicating that something is wrong: we have a problem called a *spiritual migraine* or *psychological indigestion*; egoism is a spiritual disease, a sickness of the soul.

If we wish to forget it, we have to eliminate tension. Why? Because that "I" is tension and it's not that we are *tense*, rather we are *tension*; the "I" is tension, a contraction of consciousness. Eliminating tension is the way to achieve any spiritual benefit. This is what Patañjali says:

prayatna-śaithilyānanta-samāpattibhyām

> The asana is achieved by eliminating tension and meditating.

To eliminate tension is to meditate; when we eliminate tension, meditation will gradually occur. Meditation is to relate to the limitless. There are those who translate the sutra as: "The asana is a state in which you are directed toward the limitless."

Meditation is to observe: the thoughts, the feelings, and the body... to observe the limited. When you observe, the miracle occurs that the subtle becomes solid and the solid disappears. What is limitless observes the limited; the limited disappears and the limitless strengthens. When the ocean deeply and attentively observes the wave, it discovers it as water, as ocean... The wave dissolves and the ocean gets stronger.

To obtain your posture in life—that position of feeling steady and stable that you so desire—you should not live like everyone else: with that feeling that I will be settled when I get married, when I become a father, when I get the degree, when I go to school, or when I retire. You will reach your place—stable, established—only through the elimination of tension.

We change because we're so uncomfortable: we seek alcohol, drugs, cigarettes... However, contrary to popular belief, this is not the search for happiness. Many people who go out to dance, drink, and so on, aren't seeking happiness, rather they're escaping discomfort. Humanity feels deeply uncomfortable. Sutra 48 says:

tato dvandvānabhighātaḥ

> In accomplishing the asana, one also attains immunity from the pairs of opposites.

The body and the mind are one unit: they are two aspects of the same phenomenon. Any mental situation is expressed through the face or physical movements: we can notice if a person is sad, angry, annoyed, satisfied, tired, or hungry.

The senses and the body are actually the mind externalizing itself. But the mind is movement and it's very far from the asana, as the mind *is* activity.

This is why the *Yoga Sūtra* begins with *yogaś citta-vṛtti-nirodhaḥ*, or "yoga is a state in which there is no mental movement." The pairs of opposites are the movement of the mind: seeking pleasure creates more pain; seeking enjoyment causes more suffering; seeking attachment leads to hatred.

In this way, the mind lives rejecting what it does not like and running after everything that attracts it: the pleasant, the nice, and the comfortable. It chains us to two directions that are actually one single line; it drags us away from what we dislike and pushes us toward what we like. This is the polarity in which we live and by which we are enslaved. The mind moves from one place to another seeking enjoyment and happiness: in this coffee, this person, this woman, this young man, this film, this profession, etc. Seeking movement...

But when you become situated in the asana, this movement no longer affects you. When you situate yourself in a steady and comfortable posture—through the elimination of tension—the mental movement cannot bother you. One who has been able to know the posture is situated firmly in the only place where one really is. This is what it's about: to be in the place where you are: not where your image, that product of society, is, not where your belief of yourself is, nor where your thoughts and imagination about yourself are, but where *you* are; that central axis of your existence, which is the central axis of the entire universe. Only here can you be situated firmly.

You say "my eyes, my head, my house, my family, my foot, my hand, my finger, my mind, my soul, my spirit, my brain, my ideas, my ideals," but to whom does all this belong? You situate yourself where the owner of all this is, where *you* are, not where your things are. Only there can you be established firmly, and no one will move you, because only there will you feel comfortable.

People who are situated in the posture—even if they go from one place to another—cannot be moved from the here.

They move in the here...

They live in the here...

They breathe in the here...

Because they are comfortable, nothing can tempt them with any result of tomorrow: "Do this in order to later enjoy that." They say, "No," but not due to repression, rather because they are comfortable in the now, in this moment. They live in the now, they move in the here, in the present.

A mind in which the movement of the pairs of opposites ceases, is a mind that is not. That is the path of hatha yoga: obviously, it begins by working from the physical level, but it's directed toward the soul; that is the beauty, that through the physical plane you can reach the spiritual one, and yoga brings us to what we're all searching for: our posture in life.

Discover the Magic of Repetition

October 23, 2011

On several occasions, different people have approached me, seeking advice or guidance about the problem of monotony, of routine, in their spiritual practices. It happens to many people, not only within Hinduism, but also in other religions. This restlessness emerges from various aspects, for example when teaching hatha yoga.

I learned the classical system of hatha yoga originally from Swami Viṣṇu Devānanda, disciple of Swami Śivānanda. In this system, each lesson repeats more or less twelve asanas, or "postures," in a specific order. It begins with relaxation, then *sūrya-namaskāra*, then *śīrṣāsana*, standing poses, etc., and closes with final relaxation.

Often hatha yoga teachers explain:

> I have a problem. Students stop feeling attracted, they drop my classes and go to other yoga centers where

> they teach a wider range of postures, where each lesson is different, every class is distinct… and people feel more comfortable and pleased. They stop coming to my class because they find it routine and boring. Well, what should I do? Should I include more variations?

There are many hatha yoga instructors who go to seminars or go meet other teachers, often with the goal of obtaining new techniques to entertain or distract their students so that they will keep attending their classes.

I must say that it is not simply a problem related to hatha yoga but a point related to all spiritual practices, and particularly in the West. The East and West are vastly different: for the West, routine and monotony are a problem, even a threat. In the East, however, we see monotony in every involutive path as a part of the practice.

When people in the West refer to martial arts, they think of something highly entertaining because they are accustomed to watching action films. Although if you look into original martial arts—karate, kung-fu, t'ai chi ch'uan, judo, jujitsu, taekwondo, and the ancient martial arts of India—you will find an extremely monotonous practice. One who has ventured even a little bit into the field of karate—shorinjiryu or shoto-kan—understands the use of kata. Kata is a series of repetitive movements that simulates a fight with an imaginary opponent, and the series is performed like a dance. That series of movements is practiced repeatedly: not for a day, a week, a month, a year, but for many years… the same kata, the first one. Then, when your master considers the movements to be performed properly, the student moves to the second kata. The practice of the second kata lasts for years and years and years. It can be extremely boring… a routine.

We find the same thing in art, even though it is another discipline. Usually in the West, people have hardly learned to play guitar when they begin to write music or compose songs. They just learned to play drums, sing a little, and then… their own songs! Nobody wants to sing the songs of others. People want to innovate, to be amused, to unwind, to have fun, entertain themselves. It is another attitude.

On the contrary, if we look at our disciples, like Saccidānanda for example, who is learning sitar: if one observes his entire duration of practice… years! It is a monotony that is frightening in the West. This means playing the exercises of another person: ancient *rāgas*… but very ancient …that many have already played. It is not a new song or a new melody. If you go study art in India, thinking it is a type of recreation, entertainment, or amusement, you will find yourself in monotony; you will become bored.

Spiritual practices are the same: we sing every day exactly the same songs and hymns in our *pūjās*. The practice of *japa-yoga* can be tedious, completely monotonous: one mantra, not a new mantra each day, just your same mantra. It can be:

Oṁ namaḥ śivāya
Oṁ namaḥ śivāya
Oṁ namaḥ śivāya

Hariḥ oṁ
Hariḥ oṁ
Hariḥ oṁ

Hare kṛṣṇa hare kṛṣṇa kṛṣṇa kṛṣṇa hare hare,
hare rāma, hare rāma, rāma rāma hare hare

Day after day...

Hare kṛṣṇa hare kṛṣṇa kṛṣṇa kṛṣṇa hare hare,
hare rāma, hare rāma, rāma rāma hare hare

A number of rounds are chanted on the same *mālā*, on the same rosary (as it is called in the West):

Monotonous…

Obviously, it won't be long before a Western mind will find this practice boring. More than one round… it is difficult! Thus, they tell me, "Prabhuji... How can I continue doing this *japa* round every day? Is this what I am going to do? Is this my practice? No… I don't feel connected to this, I always need something new." And each mind, each ego, thinks that it is the only one like that. "I always need something new, to change… to change." It is not that you always need to change: it is the *mind* that needs to change.

The mind needs vitamins, nourishment, and the mind's food is novelty, recreation, celebrations, revelry, parties, the new thing. It is all mental nourishment: new sensations, the new partner, the new car, the new sport, the new hobby, the new place, the new practice…

It is food because if it does not receive this and enters into monotony or routine, it becomes bored and boredom is synonymous with disappearance. It bothers us. We feel uncomfortable and ask, "Is my entire life going to be like this? And where am I here?"

"Am I going to disappear? Singing other peoples' songs all the time? Repeating them? Everyday saying *oṁ… oṁ… oṁ… oṁ…* sixty times? Sixty rounds! *Oṁ… oṁ…* nothing else...? *Oṁ* this, *oṁ* that! But only *oṁ… oṁ… oṁ*?"

You feel that you are disappearing, that you are less… that you are diminishing.

The mind feels uncomfortable. There must be something new: tennis, karate, guitar, hiking, traveling, vacations, a new job, new partner, divorce, remarriage, the new car… something new! Novelty, wild party, celebration, the constant carnival…. This happens to many people, they think, "I am sick of this monotony of being single… I must marry!" So they get married and after some time, there is repetition. Always the same person, you wake up beside the same person. You come home after work and see the same person! So, you blame the other person: "I am bored because of the other, I must change! I'll look for another relationship, or… let's do something, let's have kids to entertain us!" And here comes delightful entertainment! Watching the children, worrying about them, provides plenty of distraction. But it is not easy, so then we must amuse ourselves again, how about vacations? And that is life, the life of the mind: constantly seeking distraction and novelty.

Suddenly an ashram with a guru appears… oh! This will change everything! Now… everything new! New life, big changes, entertainment, such amusement! Going to an ashram, being with the guru… everything is different… as long as it is new! But in the ashram, if you are a good disciple you are going to follow a *sādhana*, a spiritual practice, which will lead you to do a certain number of rounds on the *mālā*, a certain hourly meditation every day. If you are good at music, if that is your talent, your service will be to practice daily and do karma yoga, which can be absolutely repetitive, like making incense every day.

Routine, routine, routine...

At some point you say, "Well, outside was better because outside, there is less routine." The world and society begins to call you once again… and you change. Once again, you will be in the same situation because, in one way or another, routine will appear. Even if you get to be president of the United States, you have to wake up in the morning… and one more war like the last one… and now there are people who want you to raise their salaries, etc. Routine...

There are people who look for a specific type of work, for example, to be a journalist, police officer, or a firefighter. They try to escape from routine, from boredom, because boredom makes us feel so small! We even associate boredom with depression, sadness, because you go and disappear… nothing entertains you… you need to be entertained!

All this relates to hatha yoga, the postures: another posture, another variation… something new. "Otherwise, I will change the teacher! Why would I want a teacher who always teaches the same?" Likewise, I change the karate teacher: "Always the same kata… one year, two years, the same kata! I want a teacher who gives me a new kata each lesson! I am tired of this one… I want a new posture, I am tired of *bhujaṅgāsana!*"

That is why teachers of music, karate, yoga, or meditation usually try to offer the sought-after merchandise because in a consumer society, everything has a price. "Either I start providing entertainment for the students, or they go. So I need to bring a new kata every few classes, a new movement, a new posture, an innovation: hot yoga, cold yoga, yoga with a Turkish bath… now I hear there is nude yoga… yoga with kabbalah, yoga with crystals... So the people will not be bored, otherwise they will leave! Something must be done…"

Meditation? If you start a course, a school of meditation, and the people sit daily to meditate, they will get bored! You have to start meditation on colors… meditation on trees, enter here and go out from there, meditate on the center of the universe, stars… something! Because the people will get bored, and then, how will you maintain the school?

However, this occurs from a lack of understanding. The East has always worked with routine, unafraid of boredom, without escaping from it. As with many things in life, we escape from loneliness and from many things that seem negative and create discomfort. Because we need to take into account that being less and disappearing, troubles the mind, disturbs the ego.

From here comes our escape, even from love. Because when loving, you disappear, you are less. Let's face it! Let's go and see what boredom is. You will discover that boredom usually leads us to a state of disappearance, and to avoid disappearing, we fall asleep, because when the ego does not want to disappear… it falls asleep. In this way it disappears, but like a fool, unconscious of it.

On the contrary, in practices such as hatha yoga, while maintaining a posture, you cannot sleep. If you are in the same posture, in the same asana, but you surrender to the repetition instead of escaping from it, a great revelation will happen.

When you are in *bhujaṅgāsana*, *sarvāṅgāsana*, or in a meditative posture, remaining upright, you cannot sleep. Same when repeating your mantra, touching the *mālā*, you cannot fall asleep, no one can go to sleep when touching and counting the rounds. You will reach a state in which you are penetrating the routine. You penetrate it, accept it, but without falling asleep.

That is why many people say that *śavāsana*, or "the relaxation posture," is the most difficult posture of all, but not everyone knows why: the reason is that it is perhaps the only posture in which there is not the slightest tension or effort. It is a complete letting go. It is so easy to fall asleep in *śavāsana*! It is an invitation to sleep, therefore, it is only for advanced practitioners. In an asana like *bhujaṅgāsana* or *śīrṣāsana*, or in the practice of *sūrya-namaskāra*, obviously no one can fall asleep! However, *śavāsana*, or relaxation, is an invitation to sleep if one is not conscious. Nevertheless, it is there that you can learn perhaps one of the most important lessons because it is the corpse posture. It is like remaining conscious while entering another dimension… while dying...

In that state, you should sit to meditate daily, at the same time, in the same place if possible, but without seeking entertainment, without looking for a God for recreation, without searching for enlightenment like a party, a carnival, or amusement. Do not seek the distraction of fun: go toward routine.

Because in the end, you must understand that the reality of your eternity will be to remain here… now… in the same silence… eternally. And if you have not experienced monotony, you will not understand what all this involves.

Many people chase enlightenment as an escape from boredom, but it should not be like that. Daily, at the same time, if possible in the same place, feel and accept that monotony, do not reject it, do not escape from it. Relax in it and fall deeply into that monotony, into the routine. Soon you will see that there is monotony but there is no boredom, you will feel that you disappear.

Only then will you meet the freshness, and I do not mean the new fashion or new song; not the new sensation that awakens the mind, the ego, your past. I mean freshness, like the spring, like the first blossom of the spring... that liveliness! They are the same flowers, but fresh. You will perceive something fresh in the depths of yourself: it is the freshness of your authenticity. It will be your spiritual spring... the revelation of your freshness... of something alive... of God...

Karma Yoga - the Art of Action

July 4, 2010

We're all born creative, but creativity can either be stimulated or repressed. Unfortunately, society—with the education it offers us—represses creativity, as the collective doesn't appreciate it; rather it only values results.

Society values efficiency, which opposes creativity, even hinders it: it values repetition, which is closely related to efficiency. In a consumer society, it is more important to produce, therefore, quality is what counts: it should be nice, durable, and inexpensive. Efficiency is related to repetition and copying; in contrast, creativity is inefficient.

Therefore, we'd say that creative people feel a certain inner inclination to take a distance from the masses because they know that creativity is for the individual; as they perceive the automation of the masses, they feel an internal need to segregate themselves from it. By becoming efficient through repetition, without noticing it, we become robots.

The familial and educational systems teach us to be efficient enough to make a living in a productive consumer society; in this process, creativity is gradually being left aside.

Thus, creativity is more related to the individual: it blossoms in the individual. We see that creative people distance themselves, I wouldn't say from society, but from the worldly noise, and they seek peace, even the tranquility that anonymity offers.

Karma yoga doesn't suggest that we stop acting or doing, nor that we renounce actions, because that is considered impossible, *na hi kaścit kṣaṇam api jātu tiṣṭhaty akarma-kṛt*. It's impossible to stop acting in this world as action is intrinsic to the human being. Karma yoga suggests that there's another way to act: stop attributing the result of the action to ourselves, and moreover, stop being the origin of the action. This means going beyond the actor—the walker, the dancer, the speaker, the artist, the cleaner—which in Sanskrit is called *ahaṅkāra*. When you transcend the actor, anything you do will be an action; without transcending the doer, you will not carry out *actions*, but *reactions*, which are very different.

To grasp this, it's important to understand something much deeper. We said that creative people distance themselves from society and the collective. But where is society, the collective? If I want to find the masses, the public, do I even need to leave the house? How many people do I need to meet to say, "Oh! This is the collective, these are the masses."

Am I the masses? Am I the collective?

What do I mean by individuality?

This story began when we were in the crib and a young, newlywed couple approached us and said, "Your name is

Michael," or Peter, John, Martha, Mary... and we accepted it. And that was not our opinion, but theirs, what they chose to call us.

Since then—from our aunts and uncles, grandparents, older siblings, neighbors, classmates, coworkers, teachers, managers, etc.—we continued collecting and accumulating ideas, conclusions, and opinions about ourselves and who we are. This is how we reached the conclusion that my name is Michael, Peter, John, Mary, or Martha; that I'm Chilean, Argentinean, Russian, or American; that I'm smart, stupid, skillful or unskillful; annoying, disgusting, important, not so important, very important, etc.

Opinions about what I am are external, extraneous; they come from other people, from the masses. They are the public opinion about what I am. This collection of conclusions is called "I."

But what do I know about myself? If someone asks, "What are you?" or "Who are you?" I immediately take out my list: "My name is Michael," "I'm Chilean," "I'm Hindu," I'm this, I'm that... On that list, there is practically nothing that is my own discovery; I'm not the authority and source of any information about what I am: everything comes from a foreign authority. It's not even what I believe I am, rather it's what they have convinced me I am and I accepted it.

When I say that creativity is of the individual and not of society, I'm not saying that creativity is of the ego, because the I-idea is the sensation of separation, which is completely different from individuality. The ego is that feeling of being something apart; it's even a sense of disconnection, of separation. On the contrary, individuality is an awareness of unity.

In individuality, I am a wave, but I feel deeply connected to the ocean. I have a form, a temporal life that begins and ends. I am in space and time, but I feel deeply that I am water, ocean, liquid... Individuality has roots and these roots are profoundly embedded in the depths of existence, of life, of the Whole...

In contrast, the ego is a feeling of separation. It's superficial because it comes from something external. The I-idea is related to others; it has neither depth nor roots. The ego is deeply interested in the opinions of others because it comes from other people and lives from them. Its life is of the other.

We want to get apart from the masses, but that collective is not out there. If I'm the opinions of all those people, then the masses reside in me; I carry this deeply within me. If I want to find the public, I can do so simply by speaking.

Your reactions aren't your own, rather the entire history of humanity is reacting through you: your entire country, your entire culture, and your entire captivity; you're a slave of nationalism, of preconceived ideas, of racial segregation, of class discrimination. Many people believe that it's what they think, but in fact, it's what they *are*.

So if all my reactions are from that slavery, then how can I speak of creativity?

As I try to liberate myself from captivity, try to escape these chains, the only thing I accomplish is a more sophisticated enslavement. It becomes a more developed, modern, and spacious prison; but it continues to be the same imprisonment. It's so difficult to rebel, to revolt. Impossible!

It's easier to rebel against a dictator, against a Mussolini, against a Mao Tse-tung; it's easy to externally rise up and start a revolution to change the government, the dictatorship, the tyranny... But religion, spirituality, creativity, is a rebellion that is against yourself and your own conditioning. It's harder for the simple reason that you are resisting a tyranny that's much closer, one that's in you, that *is* you.

Karma yoga says that you are entitled to the action but not to its fruit; that you can act but out of love for the action, without expecting a result. This is completely contrary to everything that the public, the masses, or the state of captivity, are saying.

If I like to write, sing, dance, paint, or sculpt, but I am seeking applause, fame, money, status, recognition, or public appreciation, I must be very careful, because it's possible that it is not art that I love, but the thing that the masses love. Likewise, if I am speaking or writing just for a result, for the fruit, then it's not an action, but a reaction. It's the collective, the masses in me, seeking their salaries, recognition, support, rewards, medals and all, because that is the product.

What's the problem with that? One is that by seeking the result, I'm in the future because any product is clearly found in the next moment... I can't be in the now.

Therefore, in order to act without thinking of the result, I must be interested only in what I do, and not what comes from what I do. If my focus is on the result, the process is no longer so significant.

Usually, society says that what you are doing now is not what matters, that only the result is really important. But karma yogis are authentically creative people and for them, it is the act that counts and the result is a bonus, because life is happening *now*; this instant is reality, it's not what was, or what will be. What *was* is a memory, what will be is a projection of those memories, but all of this is only imagination. All that matters is what *is*. And what *is* is the act or what I'm doing. The results belong to the realm of tomorrow. Therefore, by loving what I'm doing, I am in reality, in the present moment.

Action is so vital. It's full of that freshness that life has; it's not trite. On the other hand, any reaction is robotic; it lacks life. For that reason, it's impossible for a person seeking results to be creative; what one does will always be a reaction. The reaction isn't meaningful because the result is never the creation itself. On the contrary, an action is vital, it's relevant, because it's the creation itself... *now*.

Creativity cannot be limited to the field of art, music, or dance; rather it should be applied to any field. For example, we could speak of religion and spirituality.

Karma yoga meets its pinnacle in meditation: without a foundation in karma yoga, it's impossible to meditate. Meditation is karma yoga. Meditation is to love what you do and to be interested in what is happening now; it's to situate yourself in the present moment without seeking a result, whether it is God, enlightenment, sanctity, beatitude, mystical experience, or whatever, it hasn't the least importance. If you do nothing, that is everything! The attitude of the karma yogi, which is the creative attitude, is to be situated in this instant.

Only one who understands what karma yoga is, only the creative being who is able to act without seeking the fruit of that action, is capable of meditating. Only those who love what they do and do not do it for a result are capable of meditating; they can sit in silence, in peace, and perceive that this moment is not just important, unique, or special, but it's *all that there is...*

Your entire life is this moment: there is no past—the past is there, in the memory—there is no future, this moment is everything! Do not exchange this moment for any result of enlightenment, God, sanctity, beatitude, lights, mystical realization... Only this instant! Only someone like this can go deeply into the now.

The life of the ordinary person is superficial, each moment follows the last. In meditation, however, only this moment is important, so you dive deep into it. You enter into this instant, you don't pass by each moment, it's not one, two, three, four, five. It's one, and more one, and deeper into one, until you are united with this one; it's to go into its depths. It's this moment, there is no following moment, so there is no place for results. Only this moment... and thus karma yogis find love for their work here and now, they realize life, existence, reality... and those who realize reality, realize God.

We said that the karma yogi is creative; I would say that sanctity, or enlightenment and creativity are deeply interrelated, and all art originally comes from enlightened masters. Of course, I don't refer to the art of people who go and dance or sing for a few coins, or for fame or appreciation. Art arises from those who understand that to overcome reaction, one must transcend the actor, go beyond, and settle in the center of life, existence, of all that is, and we call this center the *Self*.

The blessed Self is one center, there is no other. It's an existential experience of bliss; you can be that center, but you cannot verbalize it, define it.

In that experience, when they open their eyes, the enlightened beings see the entire world is suffering, in misery, and people seeking something that they already are. And from their bliss, trying to share it with others, they sang, they danced, they wrote poems, they painted, played instruments, and from them, art was born.

Action and Reaction in Karma Yoga

July 7, 2010

We usually refer to karma yoga as "the yoga of action" or "the yoga of activity." However, more than just teaching what action is and how to act, classic karma yoga is a wisdom that guides us to transcend reaction or the deed at its instinctive, mechanical, and automatic levels in order to wake up to the world of action. For this purpose, it is very important to understand the difference between reaction and action.

Reaction emerges from the mind; its origin is our internal, subjective world of dreams, nightmares, chaos, and disorder. Therefore, reaction always originates in the past, because the mind *is* past; it is yesterday. Reaction comes from the world of thought, which is past. Being past—coming from the memory—reaction has no relation at all to the moment, the other person, the situation. It is totally disconnected from the now because reaction is no more than an activation of specific behavioral patterns that were acquired in a past. My father learned in his sales training course that if you visit people in their office, wanting to sell them something, it's very important that they accept you. You should look around and carefully observe what there is in the office. If you see, for example, many photographs of various places in the world, you know that the person likes to travel; if you see golf or soccer trophies, you know that the person is very fond of these sports. Then, the moment you speak to them about this sport, you're activating a whole system that the other person will react positively to and will accept you. Therefore, they will be more likely to buy what you want to sell them. Of course, everyone knows this. We realize that when we approach people, we can activate their behavioral patterns in one way or another; and this is what constitutes reaction. Thus, in a way, reaction is to ignore the present, to ignore the now.

Reaction is entirely subjective and it gradually develops within you. It can be positive, as in an attraction toward something or someone, or it can be a rejection of an object or a person. It's a feeling that, for one reason or another, you don't express perhaps because of a social reason or something and it continues to grow within you. The emotion will grow for months or even years, until it spills out like an overflowing cup of tea, without taking into consideration what is happening around you.

So your reaction—be it rage, passion, or whatever—is expressed, but it has no relation whatsoever to anyone. In other words, the circumstances, the situation, the other person, and all that is found in this moment, are totally irrelevant to the reaction. They are no more than an excuse for the reaction to be expressed. You may think, "Why is he mad at me?" "What happened for this person to express such an attraction?" But a reaction, by nature, isn't related to the other person. This is one of the reasons why a reaction has no power; it isn't something *vital* like action.

Action emerges from the moment, the present. Its roots are in the depths of existence, as it's an expression or manifestation of it. Action has the vitality of what's real; it doesn't originate in the past. Like dancing with the present, it's to be in harmony with this instant, to be in tune with the other; it's a kind of conversation with the moment. Action occurs in the present, meaning everything you do, everything you touch, will have a profound meaning because it's alive. The difference between an action and a reaction is something like the difference between a genuine, natural flower, and a plastic flower. A reaction may be pleasant, but it's always trite.

Karma yoga teaches us not to stop acting because it's impossible as the *Bhagavad-gītā* says but your acting should be action and not reaction, because reaction destroys and automates you. Reaction divides because it's nothing more than a reflection of your internal conflicts and fragmentation. Each time you react, you become a little more like a computer. You push a button and you react in the same way; years pass and you find yourself reacting in the same way in the same situation.

Reaction ages you; action vitalizes. Action is innocent; reaction is manipulative because it's always seeking a result or certain goals. In the reaction, there's no love for what one does, rather an attraction to what will result from what one does.

Karma yoga teaches that if you want to act, first you need to love what you are doing. Your attention is usually attracted toward what you love, and if you love, whatever you do will attract your attention to such an extent that the action will be more important than its result. Action is innocent because this moment is everything for it; more relevant than the result, will be the process of the work. The result can be pleasant or painful, but it lacks importance.

The reaction may be dancing, playing music, or painting, yet done while seeking the result: fame, honor, money, or success. On the contrary, action loves what it's doing: it paints because it loves to paint, it loves the colors; it dances because it loves to dance.

Reaction is on the level of a technician; action is of the master. Reaction is always seeking the "how to" with its repetitive efficiency. Obviously, when we want results, we must be efficient, and the efficiency is polished and perfected by repetition.

There may be a technique in action, but it's irrelevant: you like to dance, you have such a desire to dance that you just move. Maybe you don't know the right step, maybe you don't know mambo, flamenco, salsa, or whatever, but you cannot hold yourself from that rhythm… the passion for dancing, those drums… so you move, you get lost in the dance, and that is action.

Reaction belongs to the cold consumer world that cares about the product. Action is from love, because only when you love can you give someone a flower or a hug without seeking a result, without any interest in obtaining something from it.

The giving of that flower, that caress, or that hug, is *everything*. But if there is a motive, there is no love.

Reaction has self interest, always searching for something in what it does. In reaction, there is no freedom because it's enslaved to nationalism, to preconceived ideas; it lives within the constraints of classism, of opinions. It belongs to the collective, to society, to the masses, to the public. Action is of the individual.

So karma yoga teaches us that society or the masses are not out there on the street or in some place; that to meet with society, we do not need to go outside; actually we carry it between our ears: it's the mind. The mind is society, it's the other, the fellow person; it's what you are. As long as you live from the mind, with this idea, this thought "I" that we call *ego*... you will *be* society.

Once, a young couple approached you and told you that your name was Carl, Michael, Mary, Miriam, and you accepted it. And from there, it continued with your aunts and uncles, your grandparents, your neighbors, your classmates, your college friends, your coworkers, your bosses, etc. They introduced you to many other opinions and they convinced you that you are Chilean, Argentinean, Italian, or American; that you are intelligent, stupid, attractive, or annoying, etc.; that you are a doctor, a professor... And today, when people ask you what you are, you present them with this long list of opinions, conclusions, ideas, points of view that others have about you, but nothing on this list is something that you discovered by yourself about yourself. Everything comes from others and that's what you are. That accumulation of opinions we call "I."

So reaction stems from that slavery, from all those opinions and ideas. Action, instead, stems from individuality but the individuality isn't the personality, isn't the person. The person is that feeling of separation: it's an awareness of disconnection. On the contrary, individuality is a profound experience of union with existence, with life. Individuality is a flower of the universe, *from* the universe.

Karma yoga will tell us that you can attain freedom, or *mokṣa*, by transcending the actor (the person, the doer), without attributing the action to yourself as a person—as the "I"—and without seeking the result. It's not that you won't act, but that life will happen through you, and you'll no longer be there as something or someone, a manipulator, doer, actor, or imitator.

And when you're not there, God is there.

Life happens, life passes through you. You cease to live your life, allowing life to live through you. That's a karma yogi: a pen in the hand of the writer, a brush in the hand of the artist, an instrument in the hand of existence, of life.

Communion

March 31, 2010

Satsaṅga means "to be close to the Truth," "to associate with the Truth," "to be together with the Truth." *Saṅga* is a Sanskrit word that is also used within Buddhism in the Pali language. Throughout many religions, we see an emphasis placed on being together.

In Buddhism, the word *saṅga* is used; and in Hinduism, of course, there is *sādhu-saṅga* or "*sādhus* together." This concept is even in other religions: in the New Testament, Lord Jesus says that if there are three people, or a group of people, who meet to talk about him, there he shall be. The Old Testament speaks a lot of the united people of Israel, emphasizing the togetherness and how all the people of Israel are one. We have *saṅga* in what is called the revelation of Mount Sinai: a gathering of thousands upon thousands of people in that moment in the desert, before the revelation of God.

This satsang—what we are doing now—is not a lecture, it is not communication; it is to be together. It is not a class, as to deliver a certain knowledge is not essential here; it's not that the speaker has information to transmit and the listeners passively receive it, and afterward adopt the ideas they agree with and reject the ones they do not.

In a class or a lecture there is separation; in other words, there is no *saṅga*. In satsang, we are together. This is the "being together" that the revealed scriptures speak about; that *saṅga* between the master and disciples throughout the entire history of humanity is the togetherness in which there is no separation, and that is called *communion.*

Communication comes from the mind: it is a meeting of two intellects, an exchange of knowledge that takes place on the level of thought, of the known, of memory; it is to pass on what has been learned, which stems from the past. On the contrary, communion takes place in the now; it is from the Self; it is of the present, it happens between two hearts, two presences; it occurs in the spirit.

Communion takes place in the realm of love, although love is different than attachment. Attachment is mental love, our opinion about love, our idea about it. When we say, "I love you," or "I am in love with you," we say it according to the idea that we have about love. Deep down, if we analyze it profoundly, you will see that what we call *love* is in fact attachment, the desire for pleasure, the fear of being alone, and many other things, but not love.

Communication is based on words, which are verbalized thought. In communication, if there's a moment of silence, it creates separation and disconnection. Silence in a lecture is a gaffe. In communication, people do not speak when they are angry or aloof. That silence can be offensive, painful...

it can be the silence of disconnection. On the other hand, in communion, silence is powerful, full of attention; it is a conscious silence, teeming with watchfulness, energy, and *prāṇa*. This silence is alive, fresh... It is the silence of meditation.

What are the obstacles to really being together? They are not physical obstacles because all that is physical is more related to communication. In order to communicate, you need the presence and voice of another. Communion requires nothing physical; it is transcendental. Thus, physical distance does not present an obstacle for communion. Because communion happens very deep within, the obstacle is internal, the obstacle is within us.

If I'm speaking and you all listen while keeping your points of view, then you'll interpret what I say as an idea with which you will agree or disagree: if you agree, you'll place it in your warehouse, memorize it and accept it; and if you disagree, you'll reject it. But this causes a division: my opinions separate me from yours.

It is important to see how separation happens. The ego is separation, which consists in my internal isolation, in my ideas and conclusions. The word *yoga* means "union," "integration": religion is reconnection because we are separate.

While discussing another topic some time ago, I adopted the example of the map and territory often used in neuro-linguistic programming. It's a very simple example stating that reality is the territory, and the map is our interpretation of the territory, that is, of reality. The map is a drawing of the territory that can be helpful to get an idea of the territory, which was drawn up with information about the territory, but it's not the territory itself. Likewise, we accumulate information about reality through the senses and internally fabricate our map, our version of reality, life, the world, and other people. The problem is that, at some point, each one of us stops living according to the territory (reality) and begins living according to the map (a version of reality).

And here lies the isolation, because each of us has made up a personal map, and therefore the maps differ from one another. Each person, according to his or her past, has individual interpretations. So, the obstacle to come together, or to allow that *saṅga* to happen, is all these concepts and ideas about reality and even about ourselves.

Kṛṣṇa says in the *Bhagavad-gītā*, (chapter 18, verse 66):

sarva-dharmān parityajya
mām ekaṁ śaraṇaṁ vraja
ahaṁ tvāṁ sarva-pāpebhyo
mokṣayiṣyāmi mā śucaḥ

Abandon all types of *dharma* and surrender yourself to me... Surrender! This renunciation is what brings closeness. When we speak about closeness to the master or distance from the master, to what do we refer? With the master, we are speaking of communion, not communication. The only way to be close is to renounce: renounce my past, the known; to be naked like the *gopīs* in front of Kṛṣṇa in the Yamunā, when Lord Kṛṣṇa stole their clothes and wanted to stand before each one of them; to be stripped of your past, stripped of interpretations... That is when we are close.

The master is a presence without a past or interpretations and he is therefore a door, an invitation to be close to the

Whole. When you attain communion with the master, it is communion with the Whole.

That is *dīkṣā*, or "initiation." All that is done during initiation is symbolic of what occurs in reality: when we place fruit in the fire, we are, in fact, burning the fruits of our thoughts that we have created through contact with the now, because thought is the reaction of our memory to the present; it is memory in its active aspect. We burn what we believe, what we think, what we have concluded about everything. And we place ourselves before the master, together, *totally* united. That is symbolic of what really happens in our relationship with the master.

And there they meet each other, in communion, in satsang, two people abandoning all that can be abandoned, remaining naked, as there is nothing left to abandon or renounce. Imagine a state like this! A state in which there is no attachment to money, to your family, to your country, to the planet, to your body, to any concept or idea. What is left? Your nakedness; and only then can you be *together* with the master.

Why is it so difficult? Why, in the verse *sarva-dharmān parityajya*, does Kṛṣṇa say to Arjuna, "Fear not?" It's difficult for us to come close, to reach that intimacy and be together. Communion is very difficult for us because we are terrified of insecurity.

We feel a certain illusory security in isolation: *my* house, *my* money, *my* partner, mine! There's nothing wrong with this physical security, but what we call *egoism* is to seek that security on an internal level: *my* ideas, *my* concepts; and then I separate and isolate myself.

Why do I seek security? Because I am an idea, a thought, and I'm very fragile; the ego is disconnection and that isolation debilitates me. That's why the ego is constantly seeking security and stability in all aspects—psychological, sentimental or emotional—and rejecting insecurity. But it is in insecurity that reality is found because reality is insecure; the ego prefers the illusion of the past, which offers security, because nothing can happen in the known.

The past is predictable. The ego is terrified of the unpredictable and that is why it escapes from the now, the present, reality, because in reality anything can happen and that frightens it. The ego seeks the past. It is secure to remain in the past: it can be bad, terrible, a disaster, but it is known.

That is the philosophy of the ego: "I remain in the past even though when I was a child they threw me out the window, but at least I know it; nothing worse can happen." So I stay with my reactions from childhood and that same way of thinking and I continue seeing the world as I saw it then; and the worse it was, the more stuck in the past I remain, because I am more fearful that bad things will happen again.

Therefore, my expectations are that I will not be beaten, that I will not be criticized, that I will not be told to go to hell. These expectations stem from the past. They aren't expectations of things that I don't know: If I am not yelled at, it will be marvelous. So when I am told about enlightenment and its marvel, my expectations are confined to not being yelled at.

That search for security divides us, it makes us weak. We cannot break a bundle of matches, but one separate match is weak because division weakens. And as the ego feels weak, it seeks security and stability. That's why the saint or enlightened master stops searching for security; they do not need it because they are united with the Whole. They are free from conflict, they are at peace. And what better security is there than peace?

There are people who say that egoism is evil, but egoistic people are not bad, they simply feel so defenseless, so separated, so disconnected, so alone, that they seek security in, for example, economic stability, millions of dollars, houses, people, love; but this is never enough because they are separated, disconnected from the Whole. They are weak; they are weakness.

That search for security weakens me further because it separates me further, my opinions, my ideas: "I am a communist and I will not change!" That separates me from anyone who is a capitalist; and within my party, there are those who are more fervent communists and those who are less, and "I am one of the strongest communists!" So that separates me from the other communists. And eventually, there's no one as "ist" as I am. And I'm left alone.

"I am a pluralist." But among the pluralists, "I am the most open pluralist!" So I start to become lonely with this idea of pluralism. In other words, these ideas gradually separate me. As long as I search for security in my idea, communication is possible, but not communion. Communion happens through the master. Why only through the master? Why can't it be with any person or thing? It is said that at a certain level it can happen by means of a tree, a bird, but it will always be through some master.

The master is a door. He or she is human like you, but is only a presence that has access to both dimensions. They speak your language but have the presence of the full moon, the trees, the stars.

The master is an invitation: from your humanity, you can enter through the master. We feel an irresistible, internal attraction toward the master because we aspire to reunite with the Whole. It is not that masters are charismatic or special personalities, but rather they are half-open doors through which we see the sky. We think that the stars and the moon are part of the door and we say, "What a beautiful door!" But they do not belong to the door. And when I really get to be with the master, after throwing away my ideas and my concepts, in my nakedness, I attain this communion with the master. And then the door disappears. The door is revealed as an emptiness through which I am in communion with the Whole.

By attaining this communion with the master, I attain communion with everything. Since I'm the one who made the separation, the union depends upon me and not the master. If I don't rid myself of my accumulated concepts and ideas, then I'm separated from everything. If I burn all my past, all the known, all my conclusions in the fire of initiation, then it's the beginning of being together. I'm initiated through the master, but I find myself united with everything: in communion with the stars, the moon, the sun. The master is everywhere, in this moment.

In communion with this moment, your life will cease to be a collection of hours that make up a day or many days that make up a year. In communion, every moment will become a pearl: the moments will be drops of nectar that will make up the river of your life. Every moment is communion: we must enter into it, appreciate it, truly cherish it. Enter into communion with life, with existence. *Saṅga* is communion with God, with the Truth... satsang... together.

Repression and Sublimation

April 1, 2010

It's said that desire is suffering. This is obvious. Desire is suffering because when I do not have something—be it food, a car, a house, a person, status, fame, money, beauty, knowledge, etc.—I want it; and because I don't have it, I suffer.

Likewise, obtaining what I desire—status, fame, money, a gorgeous partner, etc.—entails an effort to maintain it, given that the relative world in which we move is temporal and transient: *"dehino 'smin yathā dehe kaumāraṁ yauvanaṁ jarā,"* says the *Bhagavad-gītā* (2.13). What begins, ends; what comes, goes; and what starts, finishes. Even if you obtain what you desire, you suffer because you must make great efforts to maintain it, so the fear of losing it arises; and evidently, if you lose it, you suffer. So, desire manifests as suffering before you satisfy it, at the time you obtain the desired object, and if you lose it: before, during, and after. Suffering, pain, misery...

That is why there are many religious people—even within Hinduism—who think, "Well, to repress desire is what's appropriate, to control it so that desire ceases to exist. The end of desire is bliss." Which is true: the death of desire is bliss; but they think that repressing and controlling desires—without allowing them to be expressed—is the proper way to attain bliss.

The *Sanātana-dharma* religion has Vedic sages called *ṛṣis*, "seers" as its foundation: the *ṛṣis* were not thinkers or philosophers, but seers; they did not think about something, rather they saw it. It's like another instrument or medium: *seeing*. Therefore, what I ask is that we *see* desire in ourselves, not that we think about it, but we watch it.

What is desire? *Sanātana-dharma* tells us that there is a process: *jñāna*, or "knowledge," gives rise to *icchā*, or "desire," from which stems *kriyā*, or "action": knowledge, desire, and action. But it's important not to leave it only at the verbal level, not just as words, but to *see* it.

How does it happen? I am in front of an object—a situation, a million dollars, a car, a cake, a sandwich—and I see it. How do I understand that it's a car, a cake? Because I search my memory bank and I see my past experiences, in which I already ate thousands of cakes and sat in different cars. That is in my memory, I recognize it: I go to what was and from there I project that past into a tomorrow, in which I see myself enjoying that ice cream, that car, or that person. There, desire is born. That's the moment in which *icchā* arises; *icchā* arises from knowledge: from the mind, from thought, from the past, from the known. And from there comes action that is motivated by desires: I acquire it or strive to obtain it.

Fear yields the same process: I see something and I go to my memory or warehouse of experiences, what we call *saṁskāras*.

I see that what happened to me caused me suffering. I project that past into a tomorrow, a future, into the next moment, and I think that if it happens to me then I am going to suffer, and then fear is born: fear of suffering psychological, emotional, or physical damage.

This must be seen. Now we are seeing; we are not thinking about it, but trying to see it in ourselves: time is absolutely necessary for feelings like desire and fear to arise: not the time of the clock or calendar, not historical or chronological time—hours, days, or years—but an internal time. What do we mean by internal time? We mean what *was*, what *can be* and what *should* or *could be*. For desire or fear to exist, this type of time is essential. Without it, desire cannot exist.

This thereby reveals to us the futility and error in this attitude: In order to stop my desires, I repress and control them, meaning that when my desire or fear arises, I simply control the action. But that does not solve the problem. Why? Because when I face that cake—or that status or fame—I project it into the future and imagine myself enjoying it, yet all I do is repress the action because of my desire to stop desiring. It is as if water would start flowing from a fire hydrant when its lid remains fastened: the water would accumulate more and more, and the pressure would increase. In other words, I create another desire by wanting to not want but I understand that there is more desire, so now I want *not to want* to want desires. Sooner or later, it will explode and not always sanely. That is the path of control without understanding, without vision.

This is a basic concept: desire creates pain before the desired object is obtained, when it is obtained, and if it is lost; it creates pain because it creates slavery to the obtained.

But the greatest damage done by desire is that it makes us exchange the reality of what I am, the world of facts, for what I could be, for what I wish to be or should be.

That is to say, if we notice, I am exchanging my reality for an illusion: what *is* for a dream. Instead, to quench my thirst, a simple and real glass of water is better than hundreds of glasses of fruit juice or banana milkshakes in a dream. Nothing that you dream about—not even God or enlightenment—can help you in the slightest. Something very simple is preferable, but in reality.

That's the great misery: to ignore reality in exchange for fantasies of the past and the future. The only real thing is this moment, it's all that exists. Those thirty or forty years of your life do not exist except in your thoughts, in your mind; they are an idea. What exists in your life as a reality, as a fact, is solely this moment.

And if we said that desire and fear can exist only in time, then they cannot exist in the present because the present is not time. Some people think that there is a present, past, and future. No, only the past is time; the future is past. The psychological future—such as hopes and expectations—is only a projection of the known organized in such a way as to benefit us; the now is not time.

That is why Lord Kṛṣṇa says this to Arjuna:

na tv evāhaṁ jātu nāsaṁ
na tvaṁ neme janādhipāḥ
na caiva na bhaviṣyāmaḥ
sarve vayam ataḥ param

> There was never a time in which I, or you, or all of these kings did not exist. And in the future, none of us will cease to exist. (*Bhagavad-gītā*, 2.12)

That is to say, we existed in the past: I, you, they, separated; and in the future, we will exist: I, you, and they. But the present is not mentioned because there's nothing to say about the present; in the present there's no mind, there's no thought, there's no *jñāna*, there's no you or I.

If you enter deeply into this moment, without living a life of accumulating moments making up hours, days, months, and years, then you will see that the other disappears because the subject-object platform disappears, which only exists in thought, with a thinker who thinks the thoughts. So, in the now, it's not that you manage to control the desires, but that they cannot exist. Just as a flower cannot grow from a rock, there is no possibility of desire or fear without time.

If someone suddenly approaches you and beats you on the head with a stick, pow! You receive it but there was no fear. Perhaps you will fear the next blow that may come but not the one you received because there's nothing to fear; you are receiving it. But if someone says, "Tomorrow I'm coming to your house and I'm going to beat you!" Oh! There is fear: "What should I do? Call the police? What can I do? Someone help me, defend me, he is a madman!" In order to fear, as well as to desire anything, time is needed: I project that blow, I see myself struck on the head, and I see myself in the hospital. Therefore, I feel fear. There must be time to fear. But in the now, there is no fear.

Many people believe that saints are very brave. They have no fear, but not out of bravery. Neither do they desire, but not because they have controlled their desires, rather because they move in the now, in the present, in which desire and fear do not exist.

In the now, sublimation takes place; it's not that desire is destroyed, it's that desire and fear cannot grow in the now. But this is a kind of sublimation because only then, situated in the now and watching, can you realize what you are actually looking for: you run for things, objects, money, situations, fame, power, status, people, but you do not actually want to collect many little, green pieces of paper with portraits of George Washington or Thomas Jefferson. When you want fame, it's not that you want to see many people applauding before you. You do not seek to be the top of the class in order to be the flag-bearer and hold a stick with colorful fabric at its top. There are sticks everywhere, and flags that you can hold in your house and stand with the fabric an hour a day if you want, and be happy. But that's not what you seek!

When we seek a bigger, new car with more advantages, a larger house, etc., what we're seeking is expansion, less limitation. In our depths, we feel an unlimited state: existing without limits, knowing without limits, enjoying and loving without limits. We seek the expansion of our consciousness, not little objects, papers, situations, and people who will feel something for me or look at me.

We can prove this because whoever has obtained these things isn't happy with them. Otherwise, people with money and fame would not commit suicide as many of them do. One who has not attained this at least has the hope to reach it, still projecting that past, saying: "But when I get it, I'll be happy." Upon reaching it, there is no future left. The person is already beyond hope and, therefore, there's nothing left but to jump off the balcony.

So, I can only desire things that I don't have; it would be foolish to want to be Chilean, I'm already Chilean! It would be foolish of me to wish to be a sannyasi, or to have orange clothes, or a beard. It's not logical; you cannot desire something that you have or that you are. You always desire what you are not: you imagine a state in which you are not, possessing something that you don't have.

This now leads you to notice that what you desire to be, you *already are;* that you *already are* where you wish to be. And that's the sublimation of desire. You are unlimited consciousness, you are an ocean of consciousness, without limits, wide, *ahaṁ brahmāsmi*, "you are Brahman," you are *That.*

And that's why I invite you to this *now.* The now is that invitation; the present is constantly inviting you. There's no need to struggle against desire and fear, no need to repress them. It should be another direction: to accept this invitation from the now that awaits you.

Each moment is an invitation to listen to these words and pay attention to that space where these words reach; to pay attention to this presence of what you are, where everything really happens, this infinite space of consciousness, which is what you really are: a timeless space. It's the now and only there do you find the peace in which there is no desire or fear, no yesterday or tomorrow, only an eternal present.

Desire

April 16, 2010

The *Bhagavad-gītā*, chapter 16, verse 10, reads:

kāmam āśritya duṣpūraṁ
dambha-māna-madānvitāḥ
mohād gṛhītvāsad-grāhān
pravartante 'śuci-vratāḥ

> [The demoniac], possessed by insatiable desires and filled with vanity, pride, and arrogance, have evil intentions based on error, and engage in labors impelled by impure intentions.

This verse is perhaps a good opportunity to continue delving into this subject of desire that we have been discussing lately.

I must always clarify that what's happening here is not a class in the sense that we are used to. This is not a lecture because it is not about instructing or teaching, or delivering information of any kind. Rather, it is what we call in Sanskrit *satsaṅga*.

Satsaṅga is a Sanskrit word that means "a meeting with the Truth." *Sat* is "Truth" and *saṅga* is "together," and it refers to situations such as associating with spiritual seekers, saintly people or being close to the master. It's to be together, to gather and somehow, in such a meeting, we perceive the Truth.

To understand the deepest meaning of the word *satsaṅga*, we must examine what it is to be together; what it is to be *really* together, not just close, not merely gathered, but together; not communicating, but in communion.

Communication occurs between two minds: it's a meeting, but on an intellectual or verbal level. Togetherness is an encounter at the level of the soul, at the spiritual level; it's a communion. To really be together requires giving up or renouncing all that separates us; I'm referring to the internal separation, not the physical one, because people can be very distant physically but very close internally. When we speak of satsang—or of the closeness between master and disciple—we are speaking of a spiritual or internal closeness.

The obstacles that cause internal separation are our various concepts or ways of seeing life. Only by renouncing these, even just for a moment, is it possible to be together. And by renouncing our ideas and being together, the Truth is born.

This is what the *Bhagavad-gītā* (4.34) tells us: in order to find the Truth, we must associate with someone who is *tattva-darśin*, "someone who has seen the Truth." In this communion, in this being together, the Truth can be perceived by the fact of being together. In other words, it's not the information that is delivered in the satsang, nor the words spoken. This isn't a meeting at the level of teacher-student; it's an encounter at the level of guru-disciple. The meeting between a teacher and student takes place on the intellectual, mental, verbal levels: communication. This, however, is communion; it's at the level of the soul, the heart, the spirit.

We said that today we were going to speak about desire. What's this power of desire, which moves and drives humanity? It's practically a force that drags us—both individually and collectively—to such a degree that the quality of our lives is a result of the kind of desires we have. Desire is that important!

What is desire? Where does it originate? Where does it come from?

All the religions, including Buddhism, Islam, Judaism, and Christianity, inform us in one way or another, of the suffering that desire entails and of the problems it leads us to.

But it's important to understand the origin of desire, since the resolution of any problem comes from our awareness of it, not from a medicine, method, or so-called solution; that's why, repressing it or escaping from it will not solve anything. In other words, the seeker of the Truth is not a solutionist.

In the spiritual and religious fields, we find solution-seekers everywhere, who give rise, of course, to solution-providers or saviors. There are people who are always looking for a way to escape misery, pain, or sorrow, so they run after the mantra, the method, or the guru that will provide the solution. However, on the retroprogressive process, for the sincere seeker who wishes to know Truth, God, love, hate, or fear—who wishes to see and become what Hinduism calls a *ṛṣi*, or a "seer"—controlling, repressing, or escaping something will not be very helpful. Obviously, when I'm trying to escape from something, I can't see or examine it. So the important thing is to try to see what desire is and where it comes from.

Lately, I have been speaking about this very interesting concept taken from neuro-linguistic programming, which may superficially seem so simple, but is actually quite useful: the map is not the territory. Reality is compared to the territory of a country or a city, and the map represents our version of reality. In other words, we acquire information through the senses—smell, sight, touch, etc.—with which we draw up an internal map and then we perceive reality according to this map.

The territory, however, is not the map just as reality is not the version that we've developed.

Maps consist of symbols: the roads are represented by lines and the cities by points, but these are not the roads or cities themselves. Likewise, in our internal map, in our internal version of reality, we have symbols: ideas, words, shapes, forms, concepts, etc. For example, money, a flag, a car... Each one of these symbols—which is a product of the past, of memory—is something we perceived somewhere; these perceptions, which gave rise to interpretations, were memorized as symbols: I see money according to my family, my city, my past, and my experiences. Money is a symbol that generates a certain feeling in me. Each symbol—the car, the house, the partner—causes a particular sensation to arise within me; someone else may have the same symbol, but it will evoke something different.

If that feeling is unpleasant, it'll give rise to what we call *fear* or *rejection*, which urges us to escape from this symbol. But if the interpretation of that symbol evokes a pleasant sensation, I'll strive to attain it; therefore, this creates the chain that, in yoga, is known as *jñāna*, *icchā*, *kriyā*: knowledge is the force that impels me, from which desire develops, and desire drives me into action.

Such an action—which isn't a free action—stems from the past and is born from desire, but that action is not directed at attaining the object itself, rather it is chasing the feeling. For instance, money causes a pleasant feeling of power in me, so I act to obtain money in order to be able to experience that feeling of power.

We all know, however, that desires are never satisfied because once we fulfill a desire, there are more desires. And when we satisfy those desires… more desires! In this manner, we will never be satisfied. We enter into this routine of satisfying sensations provoked by a symbol and this habit grows stronger insofar as we continue satisfying, but we never feel satiated.

The reason is very simple: sensations are not something substantial; they are ephemeral and they stem from an interpretation, which is ephemeral as well, of a mental symbol, which is just as ephemeral. Bottom line, it's all a world of bubbles, illusions, fantasies, and dreams; there's nothing substantial there.

Therefore, even if I turn into an automatic sensation-satisfying machine, I'll never feel satisfied because I don't have power, just a sensation of power; instead of attention, I have the feeling of attention.

For example, if I have a symbol of being a piano player or a guitarist and I imagine feeling loved by the many people paying attention to me, then that sensation of being loved makes me strive to become a great artist; then I reach that sensation of being loved, but it's only a sensation, it's not really being loved; similarly, the sensation of happiness isn't happiness, the feeling of peace is not peace.

On the other hand, I can never feel satisfied by fulfilling these sensations and desires because desire is past, it comes from the past, it moves from the past and satisfies something in the past; it's not related to the present. Therefore, desire is time: it comes from the past and projects itself toward the future. The symbol is in the memory and the feeling it produces is projected into the future: how would I see myself with this symbol, with the car, the money, the family, the medal, the diploma, or whatever? So, I run after this how-it-could-be, and whatever is not in the now cannot satisfy me: no food that I ate a year ago or will eat next year, can satisfy my hunger now. A glass of water that I drank two months ago or that I'm promised to be given six months from now, will not be able to quench the thirst that I feel in this moment.

Desire is a mechanism that's entirely related to the past and the future, never to the present; it has nothing to do with this moment. Desire drags us to renounce the present for a future; it drives us to give up and ignore the now—reality, life, existence—in order to get entangled in the tomorrow. In desire, we completely renounce what is—what I am, what I have—for what might be, what I will obtain. It's to exchange reality for a dream, a fantasy.

But one day, a very strange desire appears: a desire for peace, freedom, reality, to fly beyond what we are, it is a desire that many have termed *the call of God.* One day a desire that is different from all the others awakens, one that includes all desires within itself. The difference is that we know that this desire cannot be satisfied by trying to satisfy it. It cannot be satisfied tomorrow or in the future, so there is no need for any action that is motivated by a sensation.

It's desire for love, not for the sensation of love; it's not the desire to fulfill a feeling of freedom, but to *be* freedom. It's not the desire to fulfill the feeling we experience when hearing the word "truth," but it's a desire for the Truth itself, the origin or the source of all symbols.

Then, many people fall into the error of transforming these things—God, Truth, freedom, nothingness, the Whole—into symbols that again evoke sensations. They begin to perform different practices to obtain that feeling and finally fall into the same mechanism that we spoke about earlier, because they rely on the concept that if I desire freedom, I must practice *sādhana*, meditation, *japa*, or read books in order to be free. But, the direction is different: you *are* free by nature! Your essence is freedom itself. Yes to *sādhana*, or "practice," but only to make sure you don't forget this, nothing else.

Desire should be *not doing*. This desire for God should be allowed to rest in its origin. We should utilize it like an instrument, like a vehicle that leads us toward the origin of this desire. Because it's not that you desire the Truth, but rather the desire for enlightenment is the Truth desiring you. You should rest attentively in this desire, allow it to return; watch and observe where it leads you, where it takes you; you will see that it leads you to yourself, back home, back to the place that you never left, that you never abandoned.

Jump into the Real Dimension

February 20, 2010

oṁ
oṁ
oṁ

oṁ gaṁ gaṇapataye namaḥ
oṁ guṁ gurubhyo namaḥ
om aiṁ sarasvatyai namaḥ

oṁ saha nāv avatu
saha nau bhunaktu
saha vīryaṁ karavāvahai
tejasvi nāv adhītam astu
mā vidviṣāvahai

oṁ śāntiḥ śāntiḥ śāntiḥ
hariḥ oṁ tat sat

I called my book *Yoga: Union with Reality* because the human being lives completely disconnected from reality. We are educated, we grow up and develop in the mental dimension of ideas. Our world is a world of thoughts, conclusions, and concepts. This is why it is said that when the revelation called *enlightenment* happens, the world disappears, but it's this world of ideas that evaporates, so we cease to move in the world of conclusions and concepts.

If we pay attention, we see that people are considered successful in our society if they can satisfy their own expectations; and what are expectations if not ideas, thoughts, or imagination? All of this develops in the world of the mind. For example, we hear: "He found the woman of his dreams," or "She found her prince charming."

Without realizing it, we live in our nostalgias and memories, reacting from that past, with expectations and hopes for a future. All these are ideas that exist only in our minds and have no relation to reality. Your expectations have no relation to the real and existential dimension of facts that occurs only in the present, now.

We do not operate with the real, but instead with a fabricated map of reality that outlines a territory; but this territory is not the map. The map is made up of ideas, information, thoughts, conclusions, and all that we've acquired through our senses. We operate with the map to such an extent that for us, our own map is the territory itself, and we confuse it with reality.

Yoga is "union with reality" in the sense that its system and words and all that is found in the revealed scriptures—as well as the words we speak now—have no intention of adding new information, ideas, concepts, or a new doctrine or philosophy.

The purpose of our debate, and of religion itself, is to wake us up to the dimension of facts and reality.

In the dimension of ideas, we know that fire burns; in the dimension of reality, we put our finger in the fire and get burned. Likewise, in the dimension of ideas we speak of fear, love, anger, rage, and jealousy; now, let's see how real all of this is in the dimension of facts. In the world of ideas we speak of memories, behavioral patterns, reactions, hopes, expectations; how real is all this in the dimension of facts, of reality?

We don't understand that the transition from material to spiritual life implies exactly that: ceasing to move in the world of ideas, concepts, expectations, memories, and conclusions in order to move in the world of facts. We begin to move not in the world of what was or what should be, not of what could have been or will be, just in the world of *what is.* That's why I define meditation as "observing what is, as it is."

If you want to grasp what I mean, it's not enough to remain on the surface of these ideas; it will be necessary to go deeper into them, because the world of facts, of reality, is found in the depths.

By "world of ideas" I mean the surface. We use words without knowing what they really symbolize. Words are symbols and we often remain in the world of symbols without analyzing them deeply.

Many people believe in God while others do not, but not many have deeply inquired into what God is. Many are religious and others irreligious, but have they truly perceived the depth of what it is to be religious? What is religion? Many claim to know the Truth, but few have taken the time to deeply reflect on what the Truth is.

This is very important, especially when we try to meditate. *Dhyāna*, or "meditation," is a leap from the world of what should be or what we want it to be, to what *is*. When we meditate, we try to observe what *is*, and therefore it is very important to renounce anything that we expect to obtain through meditation. This will be essential, because as long as there is an expectation, it will bind us to the world of thoughts.

Kṛṣṇa says in the *Bhagavad-gītā*, chapter 18, verse 66:

sarva-dharmān parityajya
mām ekaṁ śaraṇaṁ vraja
ahaṁ tvāṁ sarva-pāpebhyo
mokṣayiṣyāmi mā śucaḥ

Abandon any kind of dharma, abandon any action, abandon any duty and surrender to me. I will protect you, do not fear. What should we renounce? What should we abandon? We have to abandon that which we call *māyā* in Hinduism, or "illusion"; abandon the material world in order to transport ourselves and surrender to the spiritual. But what does this mean?

We have to renounce our mental world made up of bubbles; renounce our past, that same past we project like a fantasy in the future; renounce our expectations, that mental world in order to give in, to surrender to reality, to Kṛṣṇa, to what *is*; renounce all that we think we should be because these are not only *our* expectations and *our* hopes. If you look deeply, you will notice that perhaps you wish to satisfy the expectations of your mother or father, which are interconnected with those of your grandparents, of your whole family; all this has to be renounced.

In relation to this, Kṛṣṇa says, "Do not fear." Why fear renouncing the world of ideas? What are you afraid of? Fear of what? I am afraid because this world of ideas is what I am, or at least it's what I have been convinced that I am: a name, a person, somebody.

Renouncing this mental dimension means renouncing yourself. It means to die, disappear, evaporate. And Kṛṣṇa says, "Do not fear, you are protected."

You are not protected in the sense that nothing will happen to you. Rather, there is nobody to whom anything can happen, as that somebody is actually an idea. Renounce yourself as a dream and surrender to what you really are as a fact, as a reality.

Meditation is simply to function with what *is*, with yourself here and now. This is renunciation; this is the leap. Situate yourself, be present as what you are, here and now.

oṁ

oṁ

oṁ

śāntiḥ śāntiḥ śāntiḥ

hariḥ oṁ tat sat

Desire Hides Reality from us

April 18, 2010

In this satsang, we can analyze a bit more what this desire is that moves humanity, drags and pushes us. Practically everything that human beings do is motivated by desire. Where does desire come from? From where does it emerge? What is its root? Let's not just think about it, but try to see it in each one of us.

This is related to what we spoke of earlier about acquiring knowledge and having answers, because the way we accumulate knowledge is by creating images of everything and everyone. I store any information that I obtain, hear, and see as images because that's a way of defining it. I even define people: my friends, my mother, my father, my brother, my sister, my aunts and uncles, my neighbors, my wife, my husband; I have an image of the person that can be called a *symbol*. Then, from that moment, I'm engaging in a relationship with a symbol and that's how I relate to reality.

My country, my work, my political party, and my car are all images, and primarily, I have an image of myself.

Thus, what we call *knowledge* is an immense quantity of images or symbols. When someone says, to me "United States," it's a symbol for me. When I hear, "Jew," "Arab," "black," "Chinese," I register these words as different images.

Then comes the way in which I perceive this image or symbol. Each person interprets these images according to one's life, gives them a personal meaning. The significance of money, a car—a Cadillac or Rolls Royce—a gold watch, a partner, etc., differs for each person. First, we have the perception of this image, next the interpretation, and lastly the sensation that this interpretation gives us: for one person, money can be power; for another it is security; for yet another, a partner can be a symbol of feeling loved, or having a certain position in society, of getting attention, of not being alone, and so on.

If that feeling is unpleasant, then what we call *fear* or *rejection* arises: we don't want this feeling and we escape from it. If the feeling is pleasant, we pursue it, we want to attain it, realize it, make it a reality, perceive it, and here desire is born: the desire to experience this sensation. Subsequently, action comes: the effort to obtain money, power, fame, or to be a great politician or a great leader. Every action, however, is not for the thing itself but for that feeling contained within it.

If the image of a writer, a great musician or a grand artist conveys a feeling of attention, of being loved, and that feeling is pleasant for me, I begin to write books, to play music, to paint, or dance, or whatever; I may as well want to be a politician or a businessman. Either way, I look to be in front of the public where everyone sees me and I perceive that sensation of being loved.

Although many people may believe that I love music, art, painting, writing, or literature, what I actually do is not related to that; it is related to a feeling and a need for attention and love, for human warmth.

However, since every feeling is related to time and space, it passes quickly. People go to their homes, and I remain alone, and I want to repeat it. So... another show, another song, another presentation, another book, only to experience that sensation of people clapping for me again. We can examine countless situations, but the principle is the same: a feeling that I want to repeat, repeat, and repeat.

Like any repetition, I fall into a routine, and this starts to bore me internally. And then what? There must be change! And we once again change the image, the symbol, but in reinforcing this habit of seeking to attain sensations, I am mechanizing myself, turning myself into a machine that repeats feelings or seeks symbols that belong to a past.

In some way, I go on feeling that every time I attain these sensations, I am left empty-handed. And the more I strive to satisfy my desires, the more I find myself with yet more desires, but never truly satisfied. Because no matter how much I feel the sensation of power or security in my money, or the sensation of being loved for singing beautifully or speaking intelligently, ultimately, these are only feelings.

The feeling of power is not power; the sensation of security is not security; the feeling of being loved is not actually being loved. They are nothing more than projections of symbols, of images in the memory that were captured in a past. They are the projection of a past and have nothing to do with the reality of what occurs in this moment.

Desires are past; they are a memory projecting itself into a future, wrenching us from the reality of the present. In other words, every desire originates in a past; it is the known projecting itself as imagination in a tomorrow, pushing us and ripping us away from the reality of the now.

Desire is what *could be*, not *what is*. It's what I wish I were, not what *is*. But what I wish I were is according to some information, knowledge, symbol, or idea that I captured in the past. I perceived it according to my past; it gave me a feeling that was recorded in me and projected into a future: that is imagination.

Desires live in the mind; the mind is time and time is mind. I am obviously referring to internal time, not to the time of the calendar or clock, rather to thought-time. Thought is the past responding to the present; thought is what *was*, or what *will be*, what could be, or what I want it to be, what is expected to be... but never what *is*.

We have always been told—in every spiritual path and religion—that desire is a source of pain, suffering, and misery. This is so because every time I desire, I am giving up the present for the future, the now for a tomorrow, what *is* for what I *wish were*. I am giving up reality for a dream, a fantasy, or an illusion.

In fact, if you are thirsty, it's better to accept a glass of water in the present rather than a glass of plum juice next year, or two years ago: just a glass of water, but now. If I am hungry, I need a simple bowl of soup with a piece of bread, but now! A fine dinner two or three years ago isn't going to help me, nor will a huge twenty-course lunch three years from now: it is better to have a bowl of soup or a small piece of bread now because you can do something with the present, with reality, but not with what *will be* or what *was*. Likewise, when you desire, you're shifting your attention from what is, to what you wish would be. From here emerges much of the ignorance that we have about ourselves.

We are going through life tremendously ignorant of ourselves: people do not know who they are, but know what they wish to be. It's very interesting: ask anyone how they would like to be, and they will tell you that they want to be like this or like that. Although what they are now, no one knows. We are more interested in living in a world of theories; few live in a world of facts. Enlightenment is to live in the real world; *māyā*, or "illusion," is to live in a hypothetical world, in the world of theory.

People of desires live where they would like, not where they actually live. They are not present where they are, rather where they would like to be. More so, being neither where you are situated nor what you are, is to miss life, to miss reality. You lack the vitality of being in reality; it's a disconnection from life, reality, existence, the universe, from all that is vital.

You suffer due to desires: you are walking and your senses are exposed to something—whether a million dollars, a jewel, the latest car, a romantic partner, a very attractive man or woman—and you desire it. You suffer because you don't have it; you feel that appetite, which is desire. Then you strive to obtain it, which also entails suffering. To obtain a million dollars, that car, or that partner, you must work, do, strive, and sacrifice. And if you achieve it, you might think "Now I can relax!" But no! You have a million dollars but now you have to check the news to see if the stock market on Wall

Street went up or down, if the dollar rose or fell. The peso rises! The yen has changed!

Similarly, even if you manage to marry Miss Universe, you can lose her! And jealousy is suffering. If you have a pretty wife, you may also have the fear of losing her; if your husband is very handsome, you might fear other women will seduce him. If you have a precious jewel, then you can't go out late at night, they might rob you... Suffering!

Finally, in a life as transient and temporal as this, in which everything changes every moment, even though your wife may be Miss Universe or your husband may be a celebrity, time passes and one day you'll find that Miss Universe or the marvelous movie star has gone, and what you have beside you is an old man or an old woman sleeping. You have lost it. Everything is temporal! Money runs out, cars change. Nothing remains the same.

In a totally temporal and changing reality, everything gets lost. Whenever I am attached to something, I lose it, then I suffer: I suffer when I don't have it because I desire it; I suffer when I have it because I fear losing it; and if I lose it, I suffer again! Desire is a source of suffering, not the objects themselves, but the desire for them.

What to do? There are those who say, "Okay… so I will not desire, now I will be religious, spiritual, therefore I will not desire." But to not desire is a desire, because now I desire *not to desire* desires. So what do I do? I therefore have to desire to *stop desiring not to desire* desires. Do you see it? There is no way out.

One day, a desire appears that isn't for anything specific, but a desire for freedom. Not a desire for the sensation of freedom, it's the desire for Truth. It's not a desire for the sensation of love, but it's a desire for *love.* It's not a desire to be something or somebody that would give me a certain feeling, but a tremendous desire to *be.* Simply to be! To be what I am; this is the desire for enlightenment.

It's a very different desire because it's the only desire that isn't fulfilled by doing something, or by striving in some way for success. Much to the contrary, if I follow the mechanical process explained earlier, it would only take me further away, getting disconnected from its fulfillment.

With this desire, you should not act while projecting some image toward the future: some feeling of how it would be or how you'd look. There are those who do it: when they feel this desire, they commit the severe mistake of creating an image of Truth, of enlightenment, of God; they develop a sensation toward that image, thereafter projecting it into the future, and then chasing the feeling that is evoked by the Truth, God, enlightenment; and that disconnects them more and more, and they become frustrated.

This desire doesn't aspire to an experience in the future; you shouldn't try to fulfill it tomorrow. This desire is for resting in it, now, in the present! In the present, all other desires disappear: when you are in the now, you don't desire! But not in a sensation of the symbol *now*, rather in the present, in this moment. And there, rest in your desire, and allow it to take you toward its origin from where it comes: toward that source from which it's born. And you'll see that this desire for enlightenment is a hand extended by God to embrace you.

More than a desire for Truth, it's Truth desiring you.

More than a desire for freedom, it's freedom desiring you.

It's a divine desire; it's God calling you.

Surrender to this desire!

Let it ignite! Allow it to turn into passion! Passion for freedom, for love, for Truth...

Allow it to lead you toward its origin!

Trust it! It knows where to go.

Meditation - the Path to Freedom

February 20, 2010

oṁ
oṁ
oṁ

oṁ gaṁ gaṇapataye namaḥ
oṁ guṁ gurubhyo namaḥ
oṁ aiṁ sarasvatyai namaḥ

oṁ saha nāv avatu
saha nau bhunaktu
saha vīryaṁ karavāvahai
tejasvi nāv adhītam astu
mā vidviṣāvahai
oṁ śāntiḥ śāntiḥ śāntiḥ
hariḥ oṁ tat sat

For any religious person, seeker, dreamer, or anyone who lives with a yearning for freedom, one of the most important questions is if freedom is possible. And, what does this freedom mean? What does freedom consist of?

Some people think of politics when hearing the word *freedom*. However, freedom from communism or imperialism, freedom from the Chinese, the Arabs, or the Jews, freedom from my husband or wife; all of that isn't true freedom because in that kind of freedom, we're still completely focused on our fellow man, on the other. It's an external and superficial freedom. We can call this *material freedom*.

It requires abundant introspection to understand that it's impossible to change what happens, but what matters is changing how we see what happens to us. As is often said, don't try to change the situation; change your attitude toward it.

Thus, when we speak of *true* freedom, we are referring to being free from ourselves. Is it possible to get rid of our behavioral patterns, of this mind, which is what we are, or at least what we believe ourselves to be?

The mind is made up of pain, misery, fears, ambitions, complexes, desires. Everything that constitutes it was added by others, and all this is what I believe myself to be. In fact, it is what I *am*, because according to the way we see our lives now, that is *what we are*. And the major question is: Is it possible to transcend all this mental content and liberate ourselves?

That is our world in which we move and live. Our world is between our ears. It's the mind. That is what we are and that is our reality: the reality of our complexes, our ways of reacting, our attitudes, our fears and worries. That is our world and that is what we are. Can we free ourselves from this?

Why free ourselves? Because all that is mind is limited: comes from matter, from others, from the dimension of forms. It's information received from our parents, siblings, friends, neighbors, schoolmates, co-workers, fellow soldiers, etc. Everything—from my name to the newspaper that I like to read, and my way of reacting when someone treats me with sympathy or contempt—comes from the dimension of forms, which is limited; therefore, all that I am is necessarily limited.

Being in this way, I am a limited being, and therefore, the desire for freedom is a grace. If I'm able to break free, I would be liberated from matter. Whether or not I can free myself is a very important question.

Now we can understand that nothing I do as the mind, as this content, can lead me beyond the mind. This is very important. Nothing I do as the I-idea, as the I-ego, as the I-concept can help me to transcend what I am. Nothing the ego does can take it beyond itself. And since there is nothing that can be done, all that remains is, so to speak, to sit and watch.

This is what is called *dhyāna*, or "meditation" in Hinduism, or *Sanātana-dharma*.

Meditation can only come after you experience that there is nothing you can do, that any effort will be fruitless, because every action stems from an idea, behind which is hiding a thought, and any thought or idea comes from the limited contents of the mind. Thus the "I"—the limited "I," the I-idea—cannot bring itself beyond itself. It's impossible to lift myself by holding myself tightly. Hence, nothing else remains but to watch... observe... and do nothing. And here we reach *dhyāna*, or "meditation."

But, what is meditation? It's to observe without doing anything on any level. On the physical level, action is simply the expression of a thought, a desire, an idea, so we must not do anything on the mental level: *yogaś citta-vṛtti-nirodhaḥ*. Meditation is to do nothing on the mental level, without any movement of the *vṛttis*; it's just observing.

In this observing, we observe forms and movements. This is what we realize in karma yoga: the observation of action. In hatha yoga, while practicing the yogic postures, asanas, we observe each effort, each muscle, and each tendon. In *prāṇāyāma*, we observe our breathing: while inhaling, how the air passes through our nostrils, and while exhaling, how it comes out.

In this process of observation, we gradually interiorize. As we interiorize, we notice that what we once thought was internal becomes external. What was once the closest, my body, becomes distant, becomes something, because by observing my body, I create a distance between the "I" and the body. This is disidentification. The body stops being me to become just a body. In the same way, we continue internalizing, as we observe our thoughts, then our emotions and feelings. This is meditation.

Meditation is an observation of what is, as it is, without the influence and interference of the mind. The mind ceases to be the meditator and becomes the meditated, the observed. This is a serious challenge for many spiritual seekers: how do I cease identifying with the ego in order to discover what I really am? How do I get liberated from the ego? You can't fight against the belief you have about yourself and reject the ego or reject yourself as an ego. You can't push, kick, or beat yourself up. However, if you observe your reactions, your conclusions, the movement of thoughts and ideas, and your behavioral patterns, at a certain moment you will see a very interesting phenomenon: all that you manage to observe becomes subtle, loses solidity. Every idea, every concept, every conclusion, and every thought you observe, loses its substantiality: it evaporates, disappears. And simultaneously, the subtle gets fortified: the soul, the spirit, consciousness, and observation get solidified, until you reach the final level before *nirvikalpa-samādhi*: the observation of the observer, the observation of the meditator, the observation of yourself.

What will happen then will be the most marvelous revelation: you evaporate, you become subtle, you lose your solidity. The "I" evaporates, that which was most solid in your life: I want, I don't want, I like, I don't like, me, mine. The "I" is what we fear losing more than anything in the world, that which makes us feel threatened if something or someone diminishes it in any way. And in the moment of its disappearance, consciousness is revealed in its full splendor.

A question has puzzled me for a long time. How is it that the ideas and conclusions disappear? Why do the concepts, thoughts, and the "I" dissolve when they are observed? Why do they lose their solidity? Where do they go? Why does the observation get stronger? Why does observation, which was the most subtle and the most difficult to perceive, become solid and substantial, reaching its maximum expression when the meditator dissolves? Where does all this go?

Do you know why this dissolution takes place? By observing, this experience happens: you notice that you are not the thoughts, the ideas, the conclusions. You are not that thought, that I-idea that you believe yourself to be, but on the contrary, the thoughts and the ideas are you. You are not the conclusions and the concepts, but they are you. They originate in you, they are part of you, they are you.

Just as the wave is not the ocean—as it is limited, it has a beginning and an end, it is temporal—but the wave *is* ocean because it is made of water, in the same way, you are not the thoughts, concepts and conclusions, the "I," but they are you, because when you see them, when you observe, they are revealed as consciousness.

Every thought or idea that you observe evaporates as something separate, disconnected, but at the same time is revealed as consciousness. Then, consciousness acquires solidity and grows: the ocean becomes perceptible until finally, you don't see waves, bubbles, or foam, but you see the infinite ocean of consciousness: *tat tvam asi.* That infinite ocean of consciousness is you; it's what you really are.

oṁ

oṁ

oṁ

śāntiḥ śāntiḥ śāntiḥ
hariḥ oṁ tat sat

Observing the Internal Conflict

March 5, 2010

We'll begin by explaining something about these meetings. Let us call them *meetings* because we cannot exactly call them *classes* or *lectures*. The meeting between a master and disciple cannot be compared with a meeting between a professor and a student, because these relationships are completely different.

As far as you are concerned, whether you are a student or a disciple is a matter of attitude. The attitude of students is extremely passive; although they ask questions, they simply expect that an external entity—be it a book or a teacher—will provide knowledge.

The relationship with the spiritual master is completely different. We hear from the *Bhagavad-gītā* (4.34):

tad viddhi praṇipātena
paripraśnena sevayā
upadekṣyanti te jñānaṁ
jñāninas tattva-darśinaḥ

Here it says that the master is a *tattva-darśin*, a "seer of Truth" or "one who has seen the Truth."

The relationship of the guru toward the disciple consists in showing or pointing out something. The master is a finger pointing toward a certain direction, so it is very important that disciples have an active attitude; that they always be *with* the guru, like with a guide who helps you reach a particular place and shows you what you wish to see. Therefore, you must go with the guide, be with the guide constantly.

What can help you to remain in this closeness with the master and always follow him or her? Love and devotion are what allow you to keep your attention on the master and go with him or her, *together*. For this reason, at the beginning of our satsang, we say:

oṁ saha nāv avatu
saha nau bhunaktu
saha vīryaṁ karavāvahai
tejasvi nāv adhītam astu
mā vidviṣāvahai

That is satsang, to be together; and what unites us is the Truth.

A teacher and students pursue knowledge, whereas the guru and disciples delve deeper toward wisdom. The teacher and students move in a linear direction: one, two, three, four... If you reach ten you know more, if you reach twenty, even more; when you reach fifty you know a lot, and a hundred, you know a whole lot. Nevertheless, the direction of wisdom, of spirituality, of religion, is one, more one, even more one, and then to know the one better, to experience it, to touch it, to reach its very root, its essence, and what lies in the depths of that one.

This is why you must *follow* the master, because it is a direction the mind is not accustomed to; the mind is accustomed to the surface. That's why it is very important that you try to follow me, be *with* me.

The master never asks the disciple to agree, nor to disagree. Both the acceptance of the teachings and the resistance to them will be an obstacle because here it is not about agreeing or disagreeing, accepting or rejecting, but about investigating, discovering, seeing if what the shastras say can be verified within ourselves.

Now we will talk about yoga. The meaning of the Sanskrit word *yoga* is "union." But we can go deeper into this word, as it is not only union but also harmony, and more than that, it is a process of integration.

Why is integration necessary? Because our suffering stems from disintegration; our misery and our pain come from this fragmentation that we all carry inside. So, to attempt to go beyond or transcend suffering and pain means, in a certain way, integration.

If we observe, we will notice that all disintegration or internal division leads in some way to conflict; this conflict manifests everywhere: wars, terror, crime, social struggles. We condemn crime and domestic violence, but we don't realize that we *are* the world and society, we are part of it. So, there are no condemners or condemned, but rather, all of us are part of this universal conflict in society because it is nothing more than an expression or manifestation of the internal conflict that each one of us—or the human being as something universal—carries or *is*. This has to be looked into and analyzed.

Where does this conflict, this fragmentation originate? First of all, we will say that it stems from time, and time is thought, is mind. Of course, I'm not referring to the time of the clock or calendar, but to time itself.

For us, time is what *was* and what *will be*. The past is nostalgia, memories, the known. The future is our expectations, our hopes, what is expected from us, what should be. We believe that the past and the future exist, but the future is nothing more than my expectations, my hopes, my imagination. As I cannot aspire to or desire anything that I do not know, that future is a projection of my past. Therefore, what would be left is the past. But both the future and the past are completely illusory, because what *was* is already over! And what *will be* still is not! So, neither is reality. In this way, we can see that time is thought, it is mind, it is a mental movement. But *what is* is not time. The present, the now is not time but it is timeless.

We see the fact that time is a mental movement when we place ourselves in the present, which as we said is not time; if there is no mental movement, there are no thoughts. With the absence of thoughts, the I-thought or I-idea disappears, it vanishes.

Time and thought fragment us because they create this division between what *was* and what supposedly *will be*. They create the internal conflict that we all harbor: between what we are and what we supposedly should be, between what we are and what we are expected to be, between the expectations that our family, our parents, and society have for us, and our own expectations. It is a disintegration, a division that carries a deep conflict.

Yoga points exactly to that fragmentation. And the big question is: is it possible to be liberated from this conflict? Is it possible to distance ourselves from it or somehow transcend it? Indeed, the transcendence of this conflict entails the transcendence of ourselves, because we *are* this conflict. We are thought... we are time... we are the conflict. Therefore, trying to be free from conflict is trying to liberate ourselves from ourselves.

Transcending this conflict or not entails being happy or not, because with conflict there can be no happiness. And that is why they say that happiness belongs to the intelligent ones, belongs to those who are capable of knowing themselves, knowing life, studying existence, knowing what the world is. This is because misery emerges from the misunderstanding of yourself, not knowing what life is, and therefore entering into conflicts with life.

We should observe, see, and study within ourselves, whether we can or cannot transcend the conflict that is me, that is what I am.

However, it's highly complicated to understand the conflict because when we are in conflict, any understanding becomes difficult. Conflict stupefies us. Let's say I can understand things, situations, and people, but I understand them only with my mind, for example, and I say, "Look, I understand it intellectually, but not in my heart." In other words, in being divided, a part of us is paying attention, a part but not the whole. It is not a way of paying attention with totality.

In order to really understand something in all the aspects, you must be there with your entire mind, heart, and body, with your entire being, as a whole. But being divided, only your mind is there: you understand something, but only intellectually. As the conflict deepens, divisions or fragmentations worsen, and everything becomes so complicated. So the question is, can we go beyond the conflict? Can we transcend it?

The only way of distancing ourselves, not only from conflict but from any vice or weakness, is to watch what *is*, leaving aside our fears, ambitions, ideas, desires and conflicts. It has to be pure, clean observation, without our interference, without the interference of the mind and our desires. Only then can we watch what *is*, and not what appears to us.

We usually observe but we interpret, which means that we add our own opinion about what has been observed. I'm talking about a watchfulness that is meditation. Many tell me, "Yes, but observation does not change anything. In other words, if I am stingy or violent, if there is a conflict and I watch it, the fact that I am stingy or aggressive will not change." They do not understand that if I relate to the conflict in such a way that I try to repress or change it, then I'm simply exacerbating the conflict because I'm creating a conflict with what I see. So obviously, this won't help.

Observation places us in front of *what is, as it is.* It puts us next to the doer as watchfulness is simply changing our position: from being the doer to being the witness, or rather, to be *the witnessing*, because that someone ceases to be. What you are, as someone or something, becomes the observed. The one who meditates, or the observer, is observed. You are transformed into the very object of meditation.

So we may think that nothing changes, but this is because we don't understand how we ourselves function. We must understand that only for a short while do we consider that what we have is beautiful; usually when we first get a car, we enjoy it... it's new, it's lovely. In the beginning, everything is incredible, from our clothes to our house, even our partner. What happens afterward? We get used to them. We even get used to attitudes that we do not like in ourselves. At the beginning, we see our weaknesses, we try to overcome them, we struggle, we create more conflict, and we do not like this. For that reason, what we do is simple: we get used to them and forget we have them.

Observation is an invitation to accept our weaknesses but not to get used to them. It is not about struggling with our weaknesses, but rather, watching them without allowing them to turn into habits; it is about letting them remain there and trying to understand them.

Watchfulness, or meditation, has a magic that makes all apparently solid things become subtle, evaporate, disappear. It's like an acid. Ideas, concepts, fears, conclusions, and conflicts disappear with observation. And simultaneously, all that was subtle solidifies; the soul, the spirit, love, the Self, all become solid. Meditation is that transforming magic that transmutes waves into ocean, that makes us see that after all, the wave, the foam, and the bubbles are all water; that the conflicts, ideas, conclusions, and thoughts are ultimately consciousness. So differences, diversity, and multiplicity evaporate, leading us to awaken in the ocean of consciousness, and thus, consciousness solidifies.

Self-Investigation

October 30, 2011

Why is it so hard to understand what fear is, what freedom is, or enlightenment, love, and so on? To understand this, we should see the way we analyze everything in this life. Which method do we use if we wish to know what love or fear are? If we analyze it clearly, we will see that, generally, what we do is *think* about the idea... Thinking implies a mental movement, an activity related to thought that evidently implies the past: the known, ideas, concepts, conclusions, opinions, interpretations, and all the mental material that thought brings with it.

Is it even possible to watch, *only* watch, with the aim of exploring, investigating, questioning? Is it possible to see fear, ambition, love, goodness, compassion, or whatever, if this exploration is mental? Is it possible to analyze reality if we stay on the level of thought? Thought itself is theoretical because when I think about something I am undoubtedly projecting a past: everything I have heard about this topic, all that I have been told about it, all that I have read about it, what has happened to me regarding it, what I have seen, etc.

All this past—that is a part of my thought—cannot be excluded in the moment I think about something because what I am doing is analyzing according to that past, that is why we say "to think about." That past cannot be exempt from my process of mental speculation; we are speculating and the most problematic thing is that we cannot place ourselves in reality. Rather we remain on the basis of the speculative, theoretical, the supposed, based on some past experience.

Śaṅkara suggests to us in his *Aparokṣānubhūti* (verse 11): *notpadyate vinā jñānaṁ vicāreṇānya-sādhanaiḥ...* This *ātma-vicāra*, or "self-investigation," cannot, under any circumstances, be a part of a mental process. If I want to realize, I refer to an existential realization of what I really am. This self-investigation cannot be part of a mental process. Rather it should be to watch... a looking.

This looking—and I mean looking in the reality of facts not theories—should be an observation so attentive, so conscious... completely exempt of preconceived ideas, of the past, of opinions. Observing what *is* means leaving aside what *should be*, what we *expect to be*, what is *expected to be*, or what we *want it to be* and just observing what *is*. And this is impossible while projecting a past or the known.

Just observe, look... And let the observed be a revelation. To become closer to the revelation is only possible by watching in silence... I mean the mental silence that we experience when we draw *so near* to the observed... that the limits between the observed and the observer dissolve.

Observing the Self, in the Self, from the Self, is observing the closest thing to us. It is a self-observation; it is so intimate, free of what comes from the other; deaf to opinions, ideas, and conclusions. That mind is formed by others; it is created by them because it *is* the others; it is not me, it is *them*, because in that mind there is nothing that has not been put there by others. And only by looking without an external opinion—into yourself, through yourself, at yourself—without interpretation, without superimposing, will an existential revelation occur, just a *watching*...

We cannot attempt to know ourselves by thinking about ourselves because it is by thinking about ourselves that we have created this substitute that we call *ahaṅkāra*, or "ego." This ego is not what I am rather what I think I am, and by thinking about myself I will only fortify myself as an ego or a substitute. But in order to realize existentially what I am, that must be put aside, and in this way... only watch...

Seeking the Seeker

February 28, 2010

In the beginning, we're very clear about what we want: money, home, a partner. We see it, we perceive it. As we evolve, however, what we search for becomes less clear. A person who identifies with the body—which is something solid—searches for solid things, namely objects in the world of forms. As we subjectify our search, our object of pursuit becomes more subtle and less palpable. We do continue progressing, but as we progress, it gets harder to define what we search for: enlightenment, the Self, God… but what is God?

As we search in the world of forms, all our attention is drawn toward the object. When we pursue the subjective, both the search and our attention start turning toward ourselves, toward the internal world. Thus, self-study and self-understanding become essential.

In the search for God, for enlightenment, there comes a point when we realize we cannot continue searching for something unknown to us; rather it's essential to understand ourselves first.

Because, without understanding ourselves, without studying ourselves, without becoming aware of how we think and of what has driven us to acquire our attitudes, we cannot know what we are searching for and why. So this is a very important level: understanding ourselves.

In the material search, a person often seeks only money or pleasure of the senses, something very simple. However, is there any real change if the same person becomes religious and starts pursuing God and enlightenment? One can search for God or enlightenment, or whatever, in the same way and with the same motivation and impetus that one sought money, fame, status, or a partner. But something more radical must change in us, so that we can say: "There is a real evolution!"

This elevation consists in starting to realize that it is essential to understand ourselves before searching for God. This must be deeply examined and we will see that it is related to the topic of action: all action is born from *jñāna*, "knowledge," which causes the birth of desire or fear, and from here, action flourishes.

For an action to exist, time must exist. Without time, there can be no movement. Thus, action cannot develop without time. And what is time? Let's speak about the essence of time, not the markers of time like the clock or calendar: time is thought.

If we analyze this, if we look at it within ourselves, we'll see that everything happens in the present. What *was* is the past, which is thoughts: our memories, our nostalgias. The future is also thoughts: our expectations and hopes. This is very important to understand because the present, the now, isn't time. Therefore, in the now, there is no thought.

Test it: if for a second you are in the now... there is no thought. Thought is only past.

Jñāna, or "knowledge," is thought. You may notice that knowledge is the way in which the past reacts to the present, and all this is thought. If you watch it, you will see it. We live in that: in what was and in what we supposedly should be. This is in respect to everything, to myself as well; the past is how I was, what I saw, what I thought, what I was told, what I heard. And the future is projections: how everything should be, how I should be....

From here desire is born, because desire is the projection of what I've seen: how I would look with this or how I would enjoy that. In other words, desire is also time, thought, knowledge, *jñāna*.

Am I something different from that knowledge or not? I am what I know about myself; I am, in a certain way, memory, reminiscence.

I am time…

I am thought…

I am past. It's not that I *have* a past: *I am* past.

It is no coincidence that *Śrīmad-Bhāgavatam* (2.9.10) contains such a beautiful verse:

pravartate yatra rajas tamas tayoḥ
sattvaṁ ca miśraṁ na ca kāla-vikramaḥ
na yatra māyā kim utāpare harer
anuvratā yatra surāsurārcitāḥ

In this verse, we are told that in the transcendental abode of the Lord, the *guṇas*, or "the modes of material nature," do not exist, nor does time exist. We know that when the scriptures refer to the dwelling place of the Lord—a Vaikuṇṭha, a paradise—they refer to a divine state without time. Can we imagine this timeless state, *sanātana*? It is a state in which I am not there.

In other words, in the now, not only is there no thought, but even *you* are not there. You intend to reach Vaikuṇṭha—the dwelling of the Lord—but it is not *you* who reaches it because there, there is no time, and for you to exist, there must be time, because you are thought, you are memory, you are time.

From there, fear is also born: in my memory, I have an experience that was painful and I do not wish to repeat it. On the other hand, there is desire: I had experiences that were pleasant and I wish to repeat them. If I have what I desire, I feel pleasure; if I don't have it, I suffer. Desire and fear stem from the past, from thought—which is me. Therefore, I don't *have* fear or desire; *I am* fear, and *I am* desire.

Since *I am* this fear and *I am* this desire, it's impossible to resist them, yet I try to. What do I do in order to resist fear? I relate it to something or someone because in this way I separate myself from fear: "He frightens me," "That frightens me." And this brings me to what I call *activity*: I want something and I act to obtain it; I fear something and I act to escape it.

This is the whole story of our lives and of all humanity: escape and pursue. But, are escaping and pursuing really conscious actions? Aren't these activities mechanical and robotic? It's interesting that searching for pleasure seems different to us than escaping from pain. Nevertheless, they are one and the same, because they have the same direction.

We must see this slavery in ourselves: we act subject only to this pursuit of pleasure and escape from pain, move only in one direction. I am a slave, a robot. I don't have any freedom besides escaping from what I don't like and pursuing what I do like. And that's the whole story of my life! It's slavery, suffering, and human misery. Although I never manage, I can try to repress fear, but I cannot resist it... because *I am* fear!

That is why when you are *total* in the fear or in the desire, they disappear! Because you *are* desire, the desire is not separate from you, there is no *somebody* who desires, there is no *somebody* or *something* separate or disconnected that fears.

We can see it on an individual level and on the collective level, because *we are* the collective, *we are* the world. If I hate, humanity hates; if I get angry, humanity gets angry; if I am selfish, humanity is selfish. The story of my life is the story of humanity: if I am a slave, humanity is enslaved.

And the people who are successful, what do they do with their success? They escape from pain with greater speed, although fear also chases them even faster, and they pursue happiness or pleasure with more sophistication. If you have more money, you can buy yourself a supersonic airplane, a Rolls Royce, or better drugs, whereas if you are poor, you pursue happiness with a bottle of cheap wine; but both are in the same situation.

Humanity has reached fearsome technological advancement: it keeps making cell phones and computers, but nonetheless, people aren't happy, because a slave cannot be happy. And if we cannot liberate ourselves, then there cannot be happiness or peace. A slave cannot love; nor can a slave be truly blissful.

Many ask themselves: Where is God? What is God? What is suffering? What is pain? What am I? If these questions come from this escape from pain, from this pursuit of a paradise, of enlightenment, of a state in which I am not going to suffer, then this search may be just another action that forms a part of this slavery-activity. This action limits me, enslaves me, it doesn't let me move in any other direction.

Here we must see if our search isn't part of the same slavery: does the call of the Lord come from slavery or is it a movement in the Self? Is it a vibration in the Self that urges me to search for the Truth at any cost?

One who feels the call of God in one's heart wants Truth, not only if it is pleasant, but even if it causes suffering, even if one has to cry like the *gopīs*. One who seeks pleasure is not seeking God, but rather escaping from pain. God for this person is a cigarette, a coffee, or a more sophisticated drug, but it isn't the complete liberation from slavery. The Truth liberates as much from pleasure as from pain. Truth liberates from the entire misery.

For this reason, when searching for God, it is so important to understand ourselves. Why do we search? What do we desire? What moves us toward this spiritual search? What is the motivation? Perhaps we will discover that our suffering and our pain stem from the fact that we resist growing, we refuse to mature, and we don't accept reality *as it is*. We refuse to accept that everything changes, at every instant, and that in a reality where everything changes, we can't become attached to anything or anyone, because that which we become attached to, is not the same the next moment! Places, people, objects... everything changes!

Perhaps by understanding ourselves, we will understand this flow of life, in which consciousness continues to manifest itself in infinite forms. Instead of being attached, we should learn to flow with consciousness itself and to allow ourselves to mature, to let ourselves grow, to stop resisting this maturation. In this way, our action will no longer come from a past; it will not be just a search for an aspirin or an escape from pain, but it will be an expression of that consciousness.

What is, as it is

October 30, 2011

Aparokṣānubhūti, this brilliant work by Śaṅkarācārya, states in verse 11:

notpadyate vinā jñānaṁ
vicāreṇānya-sādhanaiḥ
yathā padārtha-bhānaṁ hi
prakāśena vinā kvacit

> Just as the perception of things cannot be without light, so too, the dawn of knowledge is impossible without inquiry.

And verse 12 says:

ko 'haṁ katham idaṁ jātaṁ
ko vai kartā 'sya vidyate
upādānaṁ kim astīha
vicāraḥ so 'yam īdṛśaḥ

> Who am I? How is this world created? Who is the creator? What is the material cause of it? This is the way of inquiry.

I think that these two verses are essential in the message of Advaita, primarily because they're not religious in the sense that they neither try to convince us of the existence of a supernatural entity nor try to preach a faith. Śaṅkara isn't asking us to believe in something. These verses are more like a call to explore, to investigate, to question… And it explains that a similarity exists between exploration or investigation, and light; that if we want something to reveal itself, what we need is light, the light of investigation, of exploration.

There is so much to say about this verse! So much to understand!

Let's take the spirit of this verse, that is, the investigation that verse 12 immediately speaks about: *ko 'haṁ katham idaṁ jātaṁ ko vai kartā 'sya vidyate…* Who am I? How is this world created? So, this is the first question we ask: Who am I?

What is this *ātma-vicāraṇa*, this self-inquiry, this self-exploration, this self-investigation? What does it mean? Many disciples come to me and say: "Prabhuji, I investigate, I explore, I ask myself 'who am I?'... *ātma-vicāraṇa*... but I don't find an answer, I don't come to a conclusion."

Right now I'm an ego; a mental entity, an idea-entity, a thought-entity, because I am *what I think I am*. I'm referring to that "I" who wants and doesn't want, who likes and dislikes, whose name is this or that; the "I" who is a success or a failure; who is Chilean, Indian, American, etc. This "I" is a product of thought. It was born from the mind; it *is* the mind. It's what I think I am. So, if this search for who I am, this exploration, is thinking about myself, I'm simply fortifying myself as an ego because I *am* a thought.

This is related to the concept that we are trying to unravel. When Śaṅkara tells us that the light is the exploration, the investigation, the questioning, and then he suggests that we ask ourselves, "Who am I," that we explore "Who am I," that we investigate what or who I am, what does he mean? What does this exploration entail?

What we commonly call *exploration* is a *thinking about*. If I want to explore what fear is, I *think* about fear. If I explore what love is, evidently, I *think* about what love is. In this act of thinking—because it occurs on the mental level—I bring up all my baggage, which is the past, and all my relationships: my love for my country, my love for my parents, my love for my partner, my parents' love for me, the love of my grandma, of my grandfather, the love for my soccer team and my political party... the love that I encountered in soap operas and movies, etc. I think about what love is with this baggage and with my concept of love, which is thought, an idea, which is mental, theoretical, and unreal.

Yet the ultimate question is: is this exploration? Can this be called investigation? I think this can hardly be called questioning: it's simply the organizing of ideas, what is known as mental speculation. Nothing new can emerge from the known.

So surely this isn't what Śaṅkara or the other masters signify nor what all the religions and spiritual traditions mean by "explore." It can't be to re-order thoughts or to think about. Thinking *about* is theoretical; it's from the level of thought. It's not *real*. It's not to examine the *reality* of fear, the *reality* of love… no! It's only in ideas, in thoughts.

Therefore, is it possible to explore, investigate, question, without the mental mechanism being used, without the past, the known, or the memories intervening? If we're speaking of observing, looking, seeing "what is," without any relation to the past, we must leave aside the known, the past, and only observe what *is*. Only then will we be exploring in reality, in the facts, simply seeing *what is, as it is*... and that is meditation.

When people wonder what enlightenment is, they often come up with the following answer, "Well, I'm in illusion, so enlightenment must be the opposite of illusion!" This is how thought functions! Actually, this enlightenment—that I've created as a conclusion or an idea—is simply another aspect of slavery because everything contains something of its opposite.

All slavery contains something of freedom and vice-versa; all love contains something of hate and vice-versa. This enlightenment will contain something of illusion because it will just be a new version of illusion. It's the freedom of the slave. It's the love of the one who hates. It emerges and is born from its own opposite. This is the enlightenment of the people in illusion, the freedom of the slaves. It's not real enlightenment, real love, nor real fear!

Observing *as it is* isn't superimposing the past, the mind, the thought about the observation...

Look and observe...

Just look...

Look without interpreting, judging or condemning, without superimposing or applying, without this looking that involves your past, the known... As it is!

Near, very near... the closer you are, the clearer your vision. The smaller the distance between you and the investigated, the clearer the perception will become. It will become sharper and thus, the only thing you can *really* explore and realize, vividly and clearly, is that which is nearest to you: *what you really are...*

APPENDIX

Glossary of Sanskrit Terms

A

Advaita – Literally, "non-duality." Usually refers to the Advaita Vedanta vision that was promoted by Ādi Śaṅkarācārya, based on the Upanishads, *Brahma Sūtra*, and *Bhagavad-gītā*. It holds that nothing is different from Brahman or the Self, and that in reality only Brahman exists.

Ātma-vicāraṇa – Also *ātma-vicāra*. Self-inquiry, Self-investigation. One of the basic teachings of Vedanta (*jñāna-yoga*).

Ahaṁ brahmāsmi – Literally, "I am Brahman" (*Bṛhad-āranyakopaniṣad*, 1.4.10). One of the four *mahā-vākyas*, or Upanishadic "great sayings."

Ahaṅkāra (*ahaṁ-kāra*) – Literally, "I am the doer." The ego; false identification. It is the aspect of the mind that falsely appropriates events and phenomenon to itself, manifested in ideas such as "I" and "mine."

Aparokṣānubhūti – Literally, "the imperceptible perception." A famous book written by Ādi Śaṅkarācārya containing 144 verses, mainly dealing with the identity of the individual, the universal Self and the steps of practice toward direct experience of it. The book is held as an introductory work to Advaita Vedanta.

Asana – (1) Physical, motionless yogic posture that is stable, comfortable and should be attained by awareness, leading to the transcendence of the pairs of opposites. It has central importance in the hatha yoga system and forms the third limb of *aṣṭāṅga-yoga*. (2) seat, a chair, a place to sit.

Aṣṭāṅga-yoga – Literally, "yoga of eight limbs." The system of yoga established by the famous sage Patañjali Maharishi in his *Yoga Sūtra*. The eight limbs are: *yama* (restrictions), *niyama* (observances), asana (posture), *prāṇāyāma* (expansion of the vital energy), *pratyāhāra* (internalization of the senses), *dhāraṇā* (concentration), *dhyāna* (meditation), and *samādhi* (enlightenment).

Ayeka – Biblical Hebrew word found in the Old Testament, Genesis 3.9, meaning "where art thou?" God said this to Adam who was hiding after committing the first sin by eating the fruit of the tree of knowledge.

Arjuna – One of the protagonists of the *Mahā-bhārata*, the third of the five Pāṇḍava brothers and the son of Indra and Kuntī. An expert archer, Arjuna is considered in the shastras as the greatest warrior of his time. It was to him that the *Bhagavad-gītā* was narrated by Lord Kṛṣṇa in the battlefield of Kurukṣetra.

B

Bhagavad-gītā – Literally, "the divine song." A sacred text of 700 verses, part of the *Mahā-bhārata*, found in chapters 25 to 42 of the *Bhīṣma-parva*. Encompassing numerous truths, it is considered the most widely accepted text by all schools of *Sanātana-dharma*. It takes the form of a conversation on the battlefield of Kurukṣetra between Lord Kṛṣṇa and his disciple, the warrior Arjuna, in which Lord Kṛṣṇa explains the essence of the involutive path and the different paths of yoga.

Bhakti – Devotion, deep attachment to the Divine or anything related to God; pure love.

Bhakti yoga – The yoga of devotion. The yogic path of union with the Divine through the sublimation and expansion of the human propensity of love. Dealing with the emotional aspect, it is a process of purification of the heart and directing it to God through selfless service, glorification, prayer, worship and other devotional practices.

Bhujaṅgāsana – Cobra posture. One of the essential yogic asanas according to traditional hatha yoga.

Brahman – The Absolute, the Ultimate Reality.

C

Ceṣṭā – Movement of the limbs, motoric movement.

Cikīrṣā – Desire, the will to do.

D

Dhāraṇā – Concentration, focusing attention, fixing the mind on one point or object, single focus. The sixth limb of *aṣṭāṅga-yoga*.

Dharma – Cosmic or universal law; the essential nature or character of something; duty, righteousness, fixed law or prescribed conduct; religion.

Dhyāna – Meditation. The seventh limb of *aṣṭāṅga-yoga*. To observe what is, as it is. Observation of whatever can be observed.

Dīkṣā – Initiation as disciple according to the *Sanātana-dharma* religion by an authorized guru; a ceremony in which the guru passes along a mantra to the aspirant and accepts him or her as a disciple.

G

Gopīs – The cowherd girls of Vraja (an area of Vrindavana, India) who accompanied Lord Kṛṣṇa in his childhood pastimes. Possessing pure and unconditional love for Śrī Kṛṣṇa along with conducting selfless service, the *gopīs* symbolize a high level of divine devotion. They are considered particles of the Lord's *hlādini-śakti,* or "pleasure potency," that manifests itself fully in Rādhā.

Guṇas – Modes, qualities. Refers to the three modes or qualities of the material nature (*prakṛti*): *rajas* (passion), *tamas* (ignorance, darkness), and *sattva* (clarity, goodness).

Guru – Literally, "one who dispels the darkness." Spiritual master. One of the main principles on the way to liberation according to *Sanātana-dharma.*

H

Hatha yoga – Literally, "forced yoga." Yogic path of union with the Whole through the physical aspect of the human being, by developing awareness. Comprises the third and fourth limbs of *aṣṭāṅga-yoga.*

I

Icchā – Desire, wish.

Icchā-śakti – See *Jñāna-śakti.*

J

Japa – Literally, "muttering, whispering." Repetition of mantras, either mentally, by whispering, in a loud voice or chanting while touching the beads of a *mālā*, or prayer beads.

Jñāna – Knowledge, wisdom.

Jñāna-śakti, icchā-śakti, kriyā-śakti – The energies of the Devī, the feminine aspect and creative power of the Absolute. These three divine powers—knowledge (*jñāna*), desire (*icchā*), and action (*kriyā*)—consist in the performance of any action on the universal or individual level.

K

Kabbalah – Hebrew word that means "acceptance, reception, or receptivity." Refers to the ancient Jewish mystical school.

Karma yoga – The yogic path of union with Reality through the aspect of action by giving up the results of one's activities.

Karma yogi – One who is dedicated to the path of karma yoga.

Kārya – Action, function, act, deed.

Kriyā – Action, rite, sacrifice, religious act, activity.

Kriyā-śakti – See *Jñāna-śakti.*

Kṛṣṇa – Incarnation (*avatāra*) of Lord Viṣṇu. Appeared in Mathurā, India, to parents Vasudeva and Devakī. He also enjoyed his pastimes in Vrindavana and Dvārakā. Lord Kṛṣṇa is the beloved of Rādhā and the *gopīs*, the brother of Balarāma, the friend and spiritual master of Arjuna, and the husband of Rukmiṇī and more than 16,000 other queens. He is one of the main deities worshiped in *Sanātana-dharma.* Prabhuji refers to Kṛṣṇa as a synonym for the Divine, the Absolute, the Self, God.

M

Mahātmā – Literally, "great soul." Sometimes used as

an honorific title.

Mantra – A powerful mystical energy encapsulated in a sound vibration and composed of one or more syllables in the Sanskrit language in which the ancient *ṛṣis* had concentrated potential spiritual powers. There are many kinds of mantras for different uses and occasions. *Mokṣa-mantras* (liberating mantras) are repeated with full concentration and awareness as a tool for preparing a meditative state.

Māyā – Literally, "that which is not." Illusion, the false perception that the phenomenal world is different than the Self or Brahman

Mokṣa – Emancipation. The state of liberation from *saṁsāra*, or "the wheel of transmigration," and realization of one's true nature as one with Brahman.

Mālā – String of 108 prayer beads plus an additional bead called *sumeru*. The practitioner chants a mantra while holding one bead at a time. The beads may be made of variety of auspicious materials such as Tulasi, sandalwood, *rudrākṣa*, crystal, etc., according to the mantra that is chanted on them.

N

Nārada – Also called Nārada Muni. A celestial sage (*devarṣi*) who travels the three worlds while playing his divine *vīṇā* and chanting the glories of Lord Viṣṇu. In many sacred texts, Nārada serves as a messenger between the gods and human beings. The author of several hymns in the *Ṛg-veda*.

Nirvikalpa-samādhi – Union without alteration. The highest stage of realization according to Vedanta, in which the union between the knower, the knowing, and the known is experienced.

Niyama – Literally, "observance." Attitudes or behaviors of a practical and constructive character that spiritual aspirants should follow in the process of spiritual preparation. It is the second limb of *aṣṭāṅga-yoga*.

O

Oṁ – The most sacred mantra in *Sanātana-dharma*. Appears in the beginning and/or end of most Vedic mantras, hymns, and prayers. Described in the Vedic scriptures as the primordial sound from which everything emerges and manifests. Presented in the Sanskrit symbol ॐ.

P

Pāda – Literally, "foot." Used also to denote a section or division of a book that has four parts.

Pāḷi – The language in which the earliest Buddhist scriptures were written.

Paṇḍit – A learned man, Vedic scholar.

Patañjali Maharishi – Renowned sage and compiler of the *Yoga Sūtra*.

Prāṇa – Life force that is often referred to as "breath" or "air" because it is its most evident manifestation in the body. The energy that sustains and suffuses all processes of life in every living being and phenomenon. It flows in the body through numerous channels (*nāḍis*).

Prāṇāyāma – Literally, "expansion of the life force." A set of breathing techniques that gain consciousness of *prāṇa*. Along with the asanas, it is part of hatha yoga and is the fourth limb of *aṣṭāṅga-yoga*.

Pratyāhāra – The withdrawal and internalization of the senses, which liberates the aspirant from the control and domination of the senses. It is the fifth stage of *aṣṭāṅga-yoga*.

Pravṛtti – Inclination or will to act.

Pūjā – Literally, "to honor." It is a worship ceremony that honors the deity or the guru, in which different elements are offered such as fire, water, flowers, and incense, while chanting mantras of glorification.

R

Rajas – The mode of passion, one of the three *guṇas*.

Raja yoga – Literally, "the royal yoga." A yogic path that leads to union with the Divine through the mental aspect. It studies and analyzes the mind in order to transcend it through the system of *aṣṭāṅga-yoga*.

Rāga – A musical scale or formula for composition and improvisation in the classical Vedic music system. Each *rāga* generates a certain mood and thus belongs to a certain period of the day or season of the year. *Rāgas* have distinguished characteristics and are personified. Each *rāga* also has its respective *rāgiṇī*, a feminine aspect with similar characteristics.

Rāmakṛṣṇa – One of the greatest and most appreciated spiritual masters of Hinduism (1836-1886). Practicing various religions and paths both within and outside of *Sanātana-dharma*, he experienced the highest state of realization of complete union with Brahman, as well as ecstatic and intoxicated devotion to Mother Kālī, and was alternating between the dual and non-dual states of consciousness.

Ṛṣi – Seer, realized soul.

S

Sad-guru – True spiritual master, an enlightened and liberated being who guides disciples on the path to self-realization.

Sādhana – Religious yogic discipline, spiritual practices.

Sādhana-pāda – Literally, "section on practice." The second chapter of the *Yoga Sūtra* of Patañjali.

Sādhu-saṅga – Association with saints or elevated souls.

Samādhi – Super-consciousness or enlightenment. A state that transcends illusion and involves the absorption in one's true nature. The awakening of the consciousness to the union between the knower, the knowing and the known. The eighth and final limb of *aṣṭāṅga-yoga*.

Saṁskāras – Subtle impressions engraved into the subconscious mind, creating mental patterns of behaviors and habits. A collection of *saṁskāras* make up a character or a personality.

Sanātana – Eternal.

Sanātana-dharma – Literally, "eternal religion." Refers to the Vedic religion, Hinduism.

Saṅga – Association, company or community.

Śaṅkarācārya – (also Śaṅkara). Esteemed saint and philosopher (788 CE - 820 CE). Considered the best exponent of the Advaita Vedanta school of thought. Author of a large number of literary works, among which are the *Ātma-bodha*, *Ānanda-laharī*, *Jñāna-bodhinī*, commentaries on the ten major Upanishads, and on the *Brahma Sūtra*, *Bhagavad-gītā*, and *Mahābhārata*, as well as many Sanskrit devotional hymns.

Sannyasi (or *sannyāsin*) – Initiated, renounced monk. An ascetic who gave up worldly affairs and attachments for the sake of spiritual practice and service of the Divine. Belongs to the *sannyāsāśrama*, or the highest and final order of life within the Vedic system know as *āśrama*.

Śānti-mantra – Literally, "sound vibration of peace." Powerful Vedic prayers possessing a pacifying effect on the mind of the reciter. Each Upanishad has certain *Śānti-mantras* associated with it, which are traditionally chanted before or after its recitation. They are also found in the numerous Vedic ceremonies and rituals.

Sarvāṅgāsana – Literally, "all limbs pose." One of the essential yogic asanas according to traditional hatha yoga, also known as the shoulder stand.

Shastras – Scriptures, sacred books.

Satsang – Literally, "association with the Truth." Usually refers to a gathering of spiritual seekers, followers, and disciples with a guru, in which devotional chanting is performed and the guru gives guidance and spiritual knowledge.

Śavāsana – Literally, "the corpse pose." The relaxation posture in hatha yoga. One of the essential practices in traditional hatha yoga.

Śikṣā-guru – Instructing teacher who guides or inspires the disciple in specific aspects or phases of his or her involutive path, as opposed to the *dīkṣa-guru*, or the principal initiating spiritual master.

Śīrṣāsana – Literally, "head pose." One of the essential yogic postures according to traditional hatha yoga, also known as headstand.

Śivānanda, Swami – Appreciated Hindu Spiritual Master (1887-1963). Lived in Rishikesh, India, and taught yoga and Vedanta. Founder of the Divine Life Society and the author of more than 200 books on yoga.

Śrīmad-bhāgavatam (also *Bhāgavata Purāṇa* - A scripture of 18,000 verses compiled by the sage Vyāsadeva, dedicated to the glorification and description of the divine pastimes of Lord Viṣṇu in his various incarnations, especially his incarnation as Lord Kṛṣṇa. It is considered the most famous, beautiful and poetic of the eighteen *mahā-purāṇas.*

Sūrya-namaskāra – Literally, "sun salutation." A traditional hatha yoga sequence of 12 yogic poses, practiced along with proper breathing.

Sutra – Literally, "thread." Traditional Sanskrit literary genre of short aphorisms that contain the maximum of wisdom using the smallest amount of words. The word sutra may refer either to a single aphorism or to an entire scripture of this genre.

T

Tat tvam asi – Literally, "Thou art That." One of the four *mahā-vākyas*, or Upanishadic "great sayings," signifying that the individual self is one and the same as the Absolute Reality (Brahman).

Tattva-darśinaḥ – A seer of the Truth, realized soul, enlightened being.

V

Vaikuṇṭha – The abode of Lord Viṣṇu, a place of eternal bliss considered by the devotees of Lord Kṛṣṇa as the supreme destination of the soul that attains liberation.

Vedanta – Literally, "the final conclusion of the Vedas." Originally refers to the part of the Vedas known as Upanishads. Furthermore, it refers to the orthodox school also known as

Uttarā-mīmāṁsā, attributed to sage Vyāsadeva.

Viśva-dharma – Literally, "universal religion." Another name for *Sanātana-dharma*.

Viṣṇu Devānanda, Swami – A close disciple of Swami Śivānanda of Rishikesh, India (1927-1993). He was assigned by his guru to teach yoga and Vedanta in the West. Founder of the International Sivananda Yoga Vedanta Centers and Ashrams.

Vṛtti – Mental wave, thought.

Vyāsa (or *Vyāsadeva*) – One of the most important masters in *Sanātana-dharma*, who divided the Veda into four parts, and composed all of the main Puranas and the great *Mahābhāratha*. Revered as the *ādi-guru*, the first or the original guru represented by all other gurus, is considered the literary incarnation of Lord Viṣṇu.

Vyāsāsana – Literally, "the seat of Vyāsa." An honorific name for the guru's seat, indicating that the guru is a manifestation of Śrī Vyāsadeva, the original guru.

Y

Yama – Restraint. Referring to certain attitudes and behaviors to be restrained and avoided by a spiritual aspirant, as part of the dharmic code of conduct. Meant to purify and create harmony and peace in one's internal world as well as in one's surroundings, in the process of spiritual preparation. The first limb of *aṣṭāṅga-yoga*.

Yamunā – One of the holy rivers of India. Originating in the Himalayas, it runs parallel to the holy Ganges River, passing through Vrindavana to finally join the Ganges in Triveṇī-saṅgam, Pryāga (near Allahabad). The river in which Lord Kṛṣṇa used to bathe and play with the *gopīs* in

Vrindavana. A place of pilgrimage for devotees of Lord Kṛṣṇa.

Yoga Sūtra – The fundamental text of raja yoga, composed by the sage Patañjali Maharishi. Describes and explains the *aṣṭāṅga-yoga* system.

Index of Verses

oṁ gaṁ gaṇapataye namaḥ
oṁ guṁ gurubhyo namaḥ
oṁ aiṁ sarasvatyai namaḥ

Oṁ, salutations to Gaṇapati (Lord Gaṇeśa)
Oṁ, salutations to the gurus
Oṁ, salutations to Sarasvatī

oṁ saha nāv avatu
saha nau bhunaktu
saha vīryaṁ karavāvahai
tejasvi nāv adhītam astu
mā vidviṣāvahai
oṁ śāntiḥ śāntiḥ śāntiḥ

May He protect us both [teacher and student]. May He cause us both to enjoy the bliss of *mukti* (liberation). May we both exert ourselves to discover the true meaning of the sacred scriptures! May our studies uplift our spirit. May we never quarrel with each other. *Oṁ*, let there be threefold peace. (*Śānti-mantra* of *Taittirīyopaniṣad*, *Kaṭhopaniṣad*, and *Śvetaśvataropaniṣad*).

hariḥ oṁ tat sat

Lord Hari is the very self of *oṁ* (the primeval sound *śabda-brahman*), which is the Absolute Reality (*tat sat*).

yogaś citta-vṛtti-nirodhaḥ

Yoga is the cessation of mental activity. (*Yoga Sūtra*, 1.2)

tat tvam asi

You are that (Brahman). (*Chāndogyopaniṣad*, 6.8.7)

pravartate yatra rajas tamas tayoḥ
sattvaṁ ca miśraṁ na ca kāla-vikramaḥ
na yatra māyā kim utāpare harer
anuvratā yatra surāsurārcitāḥ

In that personal abode (Vaikuṇṭha) of the Lord, the material modes of passion (*rajas*) and ignorance (*tamas*) neither prevail nor influence goodness (*sattva*). There is no predominance of the influence of time (*kāla*), so of course not of the illusory, external energy (*māyā*), which cannot enter that region. Both the gods (*suras*) and the demons (*asuras*) worship the Lord as devotees. (*Śrīmad-bhāgavatam*, 2.9.10)

dehino 'smin yathā dehe
kaumāraṁ yauvanaṁ jarā
tathā dehāntara-prāptir
dhīras tatra na muhyati

Just as the incarnated Self passes in this body through childhood, youth, and old age, in the same way, it passes to another body. The wise ones are not deluded by this change. (*Bhagavad-gītā*, 2.13)

na hi kaścit kṣaṇam api
jātu tiṣṭhaty akarma-kṛt
kāryate hy avaśaḥ karma
sarvaḥ prakṛti-jair guṇaiḥ

Everyone is helplessly forced to act according to the qualities (*guṇas*) born from nature (*prakṛti*). Therefore, no one can cease from acting, not even for a moment. (*Bhagavad-gītā*, 3.5)

tad viddhi praṇipātena
paripraśnena sevayā
upadekṣyanti te jñānaṁ
jñāninas tattva-darśinaḥ

By humble exploration and by service [to the spiritual master], the knowers who have seen the Truth will teach you that wisdom. (*Bhagavad-gītā*, 4.34)

sarva-dharmān parityajya
mām ekaṁ śaraṇaṁ vraja
ahaṁ tvāṁ sarva-pāpebhyo
mokṣayiṣyāmi mā śucaḥ

Renounce all types of religions and surrender only to me. Fear not, I shall liberate you from all sinful reactions. (*Bhagavad-gītā*, 18.66)

notpadyate vinā jñānaṁ
vicāreṇānya-sādhanaiḥ
yathā padārtha-bhānaṁ hi
prakāśena vinā kvacit

Just as the perception of things cannot be without light, so too, the dawn of knowledge is impossible without enquiry. (*Aparokṣānubhūti*, 11)

sthira-sukham āsanam

The asana is steady and comfortable. (*Yoga Sūtra*, 2.46)

prayatna-śaithilyānanta-samāpattibhyām

The asana is achieved by eliminating tension and meditating. (*Yoga Sūtra*, 2.47) *tato dvandvānabhighātaḥ*

In achieving the asana, one also attains immunity from the pairs of opposites. (*Yoga Sūtra*, 2.48)

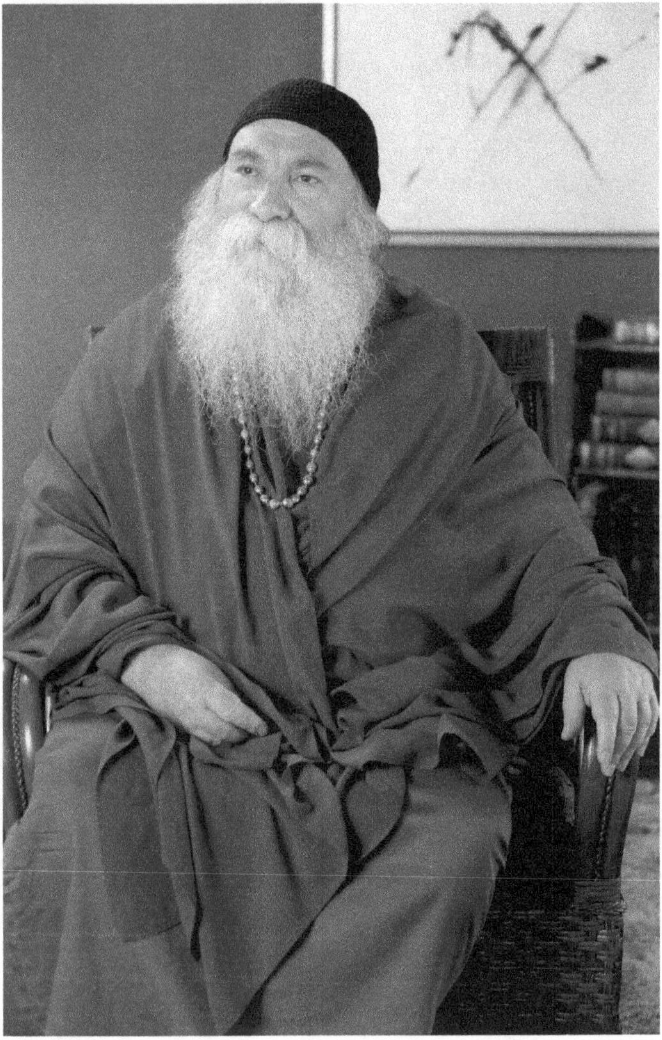

Prabhuji

David, Ben Yosef, Har-Zion
H.H. Avadhūta Bhaktivedānta Yogācārya
Ramakrishnananda Bābājī Mahārāja

Biography

David, Ben Yosef, Har-Zion, who writes under the pen name Prabhuji, is a writer, painter, and *avadhūta* mystic. In 2011, he chose to retire from society and lead the life of a hermit. He spends his days in solitude, praying, studying, writing, painting, and meditating in silence and contemplation.

Prabhuji, H.H. Avadhūta Bhaktivedānta Yogācārya Ramakrishnananda Bābājī Mahārāja, was inspired in his evolutionary process by four holy masters: H.D.G. Bhaktikavi Atulānanda Ācārya Swami Mahārāja, disciple of H.D.G. A.C. Bhaktivedānta Swami Prabhupāda, H.D.G. Avadhūta Śrī Brahmānanda Bābājī Mahārāja, disciple of H.D.G. Avadhūta Śrī Mastarāma Bābājī Mahārāja, his father, Hacham Yosef Har-Zion ZT"L, and Rabbi Shalom Dov Lifshitz ZT"L, disciple of the Lubavitcher Rebbe.

He was born on March 21, 1958 in Santiago, the capital of the Republic of Chile. When he was eight years old, he had a mystical experience that sparked his search for the Truth, or the Ultimate Reality. For more than fifty years, he has dedicated himself to explore and practice various religions, philosophies, and spiritual paths. He has devoted his life to deepening the early transformative experience that marked the beginning of his process of involution. For Prabhuji, awakening at the level of consciousness, or the transcendence of the egoic phenomenon, is the next step in humanity's evolution. He considers that the essence of every religion is self-knowledge. His syncretic vision speaks of the recognition of consciousness. Prabhuji does not proselytize. He considers any effort to convince others to be an attempt to control through manipulation.

Prabhuji is a recognized authority on Eastern wisdom. He is known for his erudition in the *Vaidika* and *Tāntrika* aspects of Hinduism and in all branches of yoga (*jñāna, karma, bhakti, haṭha, rāja, kuṇḍalinī*, tantra, mantra, and others). He has an inclusive attitude toward all religions and is intimately familiar with Judaism, Christianity, Buddhism, Sufism, Taoism, Sikhism, Jainism, Shintoism, Bahaism, and the Mapuche religion, among others. He learned about the Druze religion directly from Salach Abbas and Kamil Shchadi.

His curiosity for western thought led him to venture into the field of philosophy. He studied with his uncle, Jorge Balazs, philosopher and author of *The Golden Deer*. He also studied philosophy with Jonathan Ramos, who is a philosopher, historian, researcher, professor at the Catholic University of Salta, and author of four books: *Philosophical Revelations, Antiquity in Poems, History and Concept of Authority in Christianity*, and *Foundations of the Christian Religion*.

Prabhuji also studied philosophy with Dr. Alejandro Cavallazzi Sánchez, who holds an undergraduate degree in philosophy from the Universidad Panamericana, a master's degree in philosophy from the Universidad Iberoamericana, and a doctorate in philosophy from the Universidad Nacional

Autónoma de México (UNAM). He was a professor and researcher at the Universidad del Valle, Colombia, and is the co-author of *Philosophy in the 20th Century: A Bibliographic Map.*

Prabhuji especially delved in aesthetics, metaphysics, the philosophy of life, the philosophy of mind, the philosophy of religion, and the philosophy of being. He holds a doctorate in Vaishnava philosophy from the respected Jiva Institute in Vrindavan, India, and a doctorate in yogic philosophy from the Yoga Samskrutum University.

His profound studies, his masters' blessings, his research into the sacred scriptures, and his vast teaching experience have earned him international recognition in the field of religion and spirituality.

His spiritual search led him to study with different masters of various traditions and to travel far from his native Chile, to places as distant as Israel, India, and the USA. He has studied Hebrew and Sanskrit to deepen his understanding of the holy scriptures.

Certainly, his first spiritual master and guide was his own father, Hacham Yosef Har-Zion ZT"L, Jewish mystic, philosopher, and great Taoist researcher, who from an early age supported him in his quest. As the son of a senior police sergeant, his father grew up with strict discipline. In response to the way he was raised, he decided to give his children complete freedom and unconditional love. Prabhuji grew up without any pressure from his parents. During his early years, his father showed his son the same love regardless of his successes or failures at school. When Prabhuji decided to drop out of school in the seventh grade to devote himself to his spiritual quest, his family accepted his decision with deep respect. From the time his son was ten years old, Yosef talked to him about Hebrew spirituality. They used to engage in conversations about spirituality and religion for days on end until late at night. Yosef supported him in whatever he wanted to do in his life and his search for Truth. Prabhuji was the authentic project of freedom and love of his father, who wanted to give his son what he never had.

On his own initiative, Prabhuji began to study Eastern philosophy and religions at an early age, and to practice karate. While other children his age were watching TV or reading magazines, Prabhuji entertained himself by reading *The Tao Te Ching*, Upanishads, *The Discourses of the Buddha*, or *The Dhammapada*. During his adolescence, no one interfered with his decisions. He traveled all over Chile in search of interesting people to learn from.

It was in 1976 that he met H.D.G. Bhaktikavi Atulānanda Ācārya Swami. Gurudeva Atulānanda taught him the path of Kṛṣṇa devotion, or bhakti yoga. Years later, he was officially accepted as his disciple. He received the first initiation and the *brāhmaṇa* initiation. Finally, he was initiated into the sacred renounced order called *sannyāsa* within the line of disciplic succession Brahmā Gauḍīya Saṁpradāya.

In 1996, in Rishikesh, India, he met H.D.G. Avadhūta Śrī Brahmānanda Bābājī Mahārāja with whom he did deep studies of Advaita Vedanta and meditation. Guru Mahārāja formally initiated him as a disciple and guided him in the first steps on the sacred path of *avadhūta*.

His many teachers include significant spiritual and religious people of the stature of H.H. Swami Dayananda Sarasvatī, H.H. Swami Viṣṇu Devānanda Sarasvatī, H.H. Swami

Jyotirmayānanda Sarasvatī, H.H. Swami Pratyagbodhānanda, H.H. Swami Swahananda of the Ramakrishna Mission, and H.H. Swami Viditātmānanda of the Arsha Vidya Gurukulam.

In Vrindavan, he did in-depth studies on the path of bhakti yoga with H.H. Narahari Dāsa Bābājī Mahārāja, disciple of H.H. Nityananda Dāsa Bābājī Mahārāja of Vraja.

He also studied with some prominent disciples of His Divine Grace A.C. Bhaktivedānta Swami Prabhupāda: H.H. Atulānanda Ācārya Swami, H.H. Paramadvaiti Mahārāja, H.H. Jagajīvana Dāsa, H.H. Tamāla Kṛṣṇa Gosvāmī, H.H. Bhagavān Dāsa Mahārāja, and H.H. Kīrtanānanda Swami, among others. The wisdom of tantra was awakened in Prabhuji by H.G. Mātājī Rīnā Śarmā in India.

Several authorities of prestigious religious and spiritual institutions from India have honored Prabhuji with titles and diplomas. He was given the title *Kṛṣṇa Bhakta* by H.H. Swami Viṣṇu Devānanda, a disciple of H.H. Swami Śivānanda Sarasvatī and the founder of the Sivananda Organization. He was given the title *Bhaktivedānta* by H.H. B.A. Paramadvaiti Mahārāja, the founder of Vrinda. He was given the title *Yogācārya* by H.H. Swami Viṣṇu Devānanda, the Paramanand Institute of Yoga Sciences and Research of Indore, India, the International Yoga Federation, the Indian Association of Yoga, and the Shri Shankarananda Yogashram of Mysore, India. On March 21, 2021, he received the respectable title *Śrī Śrī Rādhā Śyam Sunder Pāda-Padma Bhakta Śiromaṇi* directly from H.H. Satyanārāyaṇa Dāsa Bābājī Mahant of the Chatu Vaiṣṇava Saṁpradāya. This title was given to him by the honorable Jiva Institute in Vrindavan, India.

The *sannyāsa* initiation was given to him by H.H. Swami

Jyotirmayānanda Sarasvatī, the founder of the Yoga Research Foundation, H.H. Kīrtanānanda Swami, H.H. B.A. Paramadvaiti Mahārāja, and H.H. Bhaktivedānta Atulānanda Ācārya. Finally, in 2011, he renounced the *sannyāsa* in order to be initiated into the highly elevated order *avadhūta bābājī* directly by his Guru Mahārāja, His Holiness Śrī Brahmānanda Bābājī Mahārāja, thus becoming part of an ancient disciplic line of *avadhūtas.* A few months before leaving his body, his spiritual master appointed him Master Ācārya, empowering him to continue the millennial *avadhūtas paramparā*, or line of disciplic succession. With this appointment, Prabhuji is the official representative of the line of this disciplic succession for the present generation.

Prabhuji spent more than forty years studying hatha yoga with prestigious masters in the field of classical and traditional yoga, such as H.H. Bapuji, H.H. Swami Viṣṇu Devānanda Sarasvatī, H.H. Swami Jyotirmayānanda Sarasvatī, H.H. Swami Satchidananda Sarasvatī, H.H. Swami Vignanananda Sarasvatī, and Śrī Madana-mohana.

He attended several systematic hatha yoga teacher training courses at prestigious institutions until he achieved the level of Master Ācārya. He has finished studies at the following institutions: the Sivananda Yoga Vedanta, the Ananda Ashram, the Yoga Research Foundation, the Integral Yoga Academy, the Patanjala Yoga Kendra, the Ma Yoga Shakti International Mission, the Prana Yoga Organization, the Rishikesh Yoga Peeth, the Swami Sivananda Yoga Research Center, and the Swami Sivananda Yogasana Research Center.

Prabhuji is a member of the Indian Association of Yoga, Yoga Alliance ERYT 500 and YACEP, the International

Association of Yoga Therapists, and the International Yoga Federation. In 2014, the International Yoga Federation honored him with the position of Honorary Member of the World Yoga Council.

His interest in the complex anatomy of the human body led him to study chiropractic at the prestigious Institute of Health of the Back and Extremities in Tel Aviv, Israel. In 1993, he received a diploma from Dr. Sheinerman, the founder and director of the institute. Later, he earned a massage therapist diploma at the Academy of Western Galilee. The knowledge acquired in this field deepened his understanding of hatha yoga and contributed to the creation of his own method.

Bhāvātīta-caitanyam Yoga is the result of efforts to improve his own practice and teaching. It is a system based solely on the teachings of his gurus and the sacred scriptures. Prabhuji has systematized different traditional yoga techniques to create a methodology suitable for the Western public. Bhāvātīta-caitanyam Yoga aims for experiencing our true nature. It promotes balance, health, and flexibility through proper diet, cleansing techniques, preparations (*āyojanas*), sequences (*vinyāsas*), postures (asanas), breathing exercises (*prāṇayama*), relaxation (*śavāsana*), meditation (*dhyāna*), and locks (*bandhas*) and seals (*mudras*) to direct and empower *prāṇa*.

Since his childhood and throughout his life, Prabhuji has been an enthusiastic admirer, student, and practitioner of classic karate-do. From the age of 13, he studied different styles in Chile, such as kenpo and kung-fu, but specialized in the most traditional Japanese style of Shotokan. He received the rank of black belt (third dan) from Shihan Kenneth Funakoshi (ninth dan). He also learned from Sensei Takahashi (seventh dan) and practiced Shorin Ryu style with Sensei Enrique Daniel Welcher (seventh dan), who granted him the rank of black belt (second dan). Through karate-do, he delved into Buddhism and gained additional knowledge about the physics of motion. Prabhuji is a member of the Funakoshi's Shotokan Karate Association.

He grew up in an artistic environment. His father, the renowned Chilean painter Hacham Yosef Har-Zion ZT"L, motivated him to devote himself to art from an early age. Thus, Prabhuji's love for painting was developed from a young age. His abstract paintings reflect the depths of the spirit.

From his earliest childhood, he has been especially attracted to and curious about postal stamps, postcards, mailboxes, postal transportation systems, and all mail-related activities. During his life, he has delved into the study of philately and has taken every opportunity to visit post offices in different cities and countries. This interest and passion transformed him into a professional philatelist, a stamp distributor authorized by the American Philatelic Society, and a member of the following societies: the Royal Philatelic Society London, the Royal Philatelic Society of Victoria, the United States Stamp Society, the Great Britain Philatelic Society, the American Philatelic Society, the Society of Israel Philatelists, the Society for Hungarian Philately, the National Philatelic Society UK, the Fort Orange Stamp Club, the American Stamp Dealers Association, the US Philatelic Classics Society, and FILABRAS – Associação dos Filatelistas Brasileiros. Based on his knowledge of philately and his extensive wisdom in theology and oriental philosophy, he created Meditative Philately or Philatelic Yoga.

For many years he lived in Israel, where he deepened his studies in Hebrew and Judaism. One of his main masters and sources of inspiration was Rabbi Shalom Dov Lifshitz ZT"L, whom he met in 1997. The great saint guided him for several years in the intricate paths of the Torah and Chassidism. The two developed a very intimate and deep relationship. In addition, Prabhuji studied the Talmud with Rabbi Raphael Rapaport Shlit"a (Ponovich), Chassidism with Rabbi Israel Lifshitz Shlit"a, and delved into the Torah with Rabbi Daniel Sandler Shlit"a. Prabhuji is a great devotee of Rabbi Mordechai Eliyahu ZT "L, by whom he was personally blessed.

The Prabhuji Mission was founded in 2003 with the aim of preserving his vision and literary work. For fifteen years (1995–2010), Prabhuji accepted a few monastic disciples who expressly requested to be initiated. In 2010, he stopped accepting monastic disciples, followers, devotees, or visitors. Currently, he only guides a small number of serious disciples who have decided to stay with their master.

In 2011, the Prabhuji Ashram (monastery) was founded in the Catskills Mountains in Upstate New York, USA. The Prabhuji Ashram is the headquarters of the Prabhuji Mission and the hermitage of Prabhuji and his monastic disciples. The ashram organizes humanitarian projects such as the Prabhuji Food Distribution Program and the Prabhuji Toy Distribution Program. Prabhuji operates various humanitarian projects, inspired in his experience that "to serve the part is to serve the Whole."

In January 2012, Prabhuji's health forced him to officially renounce public life and stop managing the mission. Since then, he has lived in solitude, completely away from the public, writing and absorbed in contemplation. He shares his experience and wisdom in books and filmed talks. His message does not promote collective spirituality, but individual and inner searching.

Prabhuji is a respected member of the American Philosophical Association, the American Association of Philosophy Teachers, the American Association of University Professors, the Southwestern Philosophical Society, the Authors Guild, the National Writers Union, PEN America, the International Writers Association, the National Association of Independent Writers and Editors, and the National Writers Association.

Prabhuji's vast literary contribution includes books in Spanish, English, and Hebrew, including *Kundalini Yoga: The Power is in you*, *What is, as it is*, *Bhakti-Yoga: The Path of Love*, *Tantra: Liberation in the World*, *Experimenting with the Truth*, *Advaita Vedanta: Be the Self*, commentaries on the *Īśāvāsya Upanishad* and the *Diamond Sūtra*, and others.

About the Prabhuji Mission

The Prabhuji Mission, founded by David, Ben Yosef, Har-Zion, is a nonprofit organization with no aim to proselytize. Its main purpose is to preserve Prabhuji's literary legacy, his teachings, vision, and message, the path of Transcendental Consciousness.

The vision of Prabhuji advocates the global awakening of consciousness, which is for him the essence of every religion, as the radical solution to all the problems of the world.

The main activities of the mission are to offer worship services, to publish Prabhuji's books, and to distribute food to people in need. All this is possible thanks to the efforts and collaboration of volunteers.

The mission no longer accepts new monastic residents.

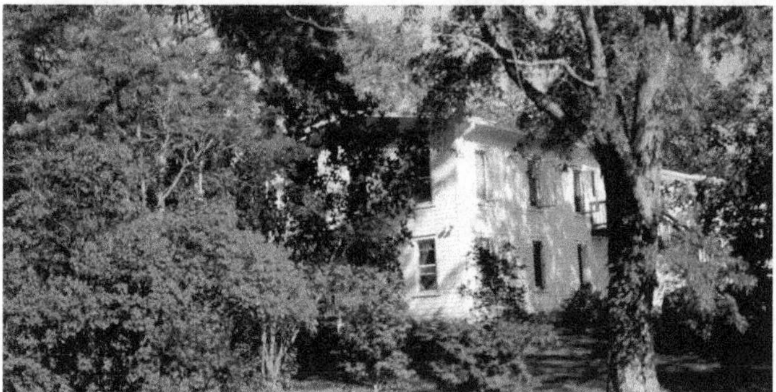

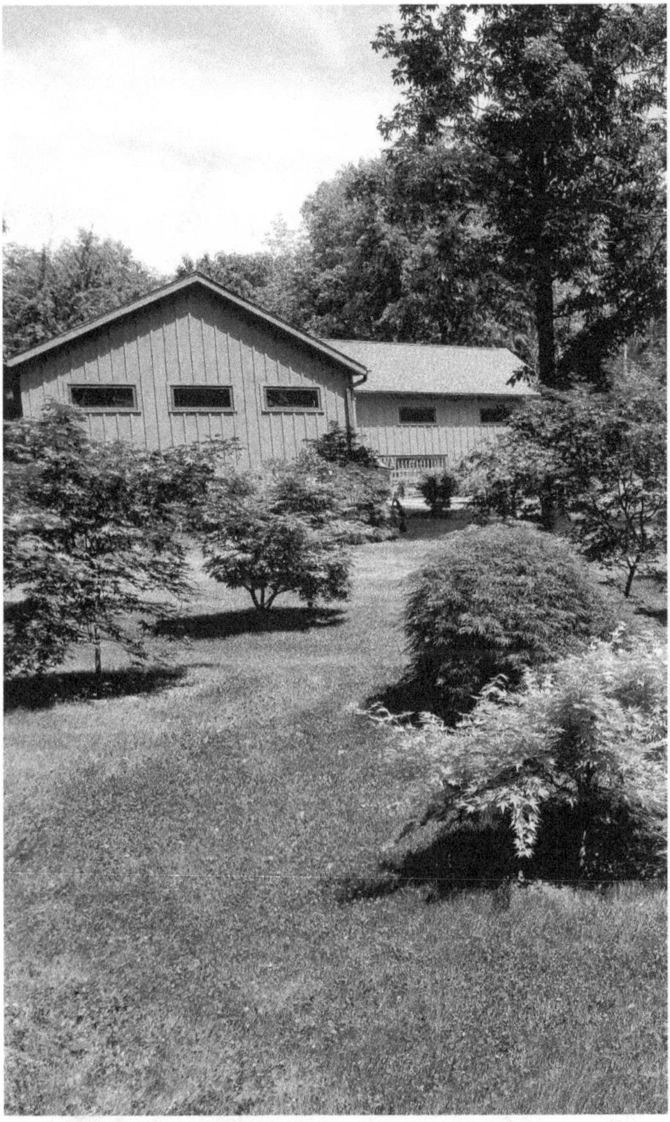

Prabhuji Ashram
Round Top, NY, USA

About the Prabhuji Ashram

The Prabhuji Ashram (monastery) was founded by Prabhuji in the Catskills Mountains in New York, USA.

It is the headquarters of the Prabhuji Mission and the hermitage of Prabhuji and his monastic disciples. It organizes humanitarian projects such as the Prabhuji Food Distribution Program and the Prabhuji Toy Distribution Program.

The Prabhuji Ashram is non-commercial and operates without soliciting donations or contributions. Its activities are funded by Prabhuji's Gifts, a non-profit company founded by Prabhuji, which sells esoteric items from different traditions that he himself has used for spiritual practices during his evolutionary process. Its mission is to preserve and disseminate traditional religious, mystical, and ancestral crafts, as well as to distribute spiritual books.

The path of Transcendental Consciousness

The path of Transcendental Consciousness does not offer methods or techniques. Nor does it list a set of obligations and restrictions. It does not require being part of a group or becoming a member of an organization, institution, society, congregation, club, or exclusive community. Living in a temple, monastery, or *āśram* is not mandatory, because it is not about a change of residence, but of consciousness. It does not require accepting any kind of authority, leader, preceptor, counselor, guide, master, or guru. It does not urge you to believe, but to doubt. It does not demand from you to accept, but to explore, investigate, examine, inquire, and question everything. It does not suggest being as you should but being what you really are.

The path of Transcendental Consciousness supports freedom of expression, but not proselytizing, because it considers preaching to be an attempt to control others through coercive manipulation. This route does not promise answers to our questions but induces us to question our answers. It does not promise to be what we are not or to attain what we have not achieved. It is a retroprogressive path of self-discovery that leads from what we think we are to what we really are. It is not the only way, nor the best, nor the simplest, superior or most direct way, but is an involutionary process par excellence that shows what is obvious and undeniable but usually goes unnoticed: that which is simple, innocent, and natural. It is a path that begins and ends in you.

Transcendental Consciousness is a continuous revelation that eternally broadens and deepens. Without being a religion, we find it in the essence of every religion and spiritual path. It is the discovery of diversity as a unique and inclusive reality. It is the encounter of consciousness with itself, aware of itself and its own reality. In fact, this path is a simple invitation to dance in the now, to love the present moment, to celebrate our authenticity, to stop living as a victim of circumstance in order to live as a passionate adventurer. It is an unconditional proposition to enter the fire of life that can only consumes dreams, illusions, and fantasies, without affecting what we are. It is a call to return to the place we have never left, without offering anything we do not possess, nor teaching anything we do not already know. It is a call for an inner revolution. It does not help us reach our desired goal, but rather prepares us for the unexpected miracle.

This path was nurtured during a life dedicated to the search for Truth. It is a grateful offering to existence for what has been received. But remember, do not look for me. Look for yourself. It is not me you need, because you are the only one that really matters. This life is just a wonderful parenthesis in eternity so you can know and love. What you long for lies in you, here and now, as what you are.

Your unconditional well-wisher,
Prabhuji

Important clarification

In 2011, Prabhuji chose to retire from society and lead a silent and contemplative life as a hermit. He spends his days in solitude, writing, painting, praying, and meditating.

Prabhuji does not accept the role of a religious authority figure that people have been trying for years to attribute to him. Although many recognize him as an enlightened being, Prabhuji does not accept to be considered a preacher, guide, coach, content creator, influencer, preceptor, mentor, counselor, consultant, monitor, tutor, teacher, instructor, educator, enlightener, pedagogue, evangelist, rabbi, *posek halacha*, healer, therapist, satsangist, psychic, leader, medium, savior, or guru. He has retired from all public activity and does not offer *sat-saṅgs*, lectures, gatherings, retreats, seminars, meetings, study groups, or courses.

For 15 years (1995–2010), Prabhuji accepted the requests of a few people who expressly asked to become disciples. In 2010, he took the irrevocable decision to refuse any further requests. He objects to social, organized, or community religiosity. His message does not promote group or collective spirituality, but individual, private, and intimate searching.

Prabhuji does not proselytize. Through his statements, he does not try to persuade, convince, or make anyone change their perspective, philosophy, or religion. Prabhuji shares his message fraternally with no intention of attracting disciples, visitors, or followers. Prabhuji does not offer advice, counseling, guidance, self-help methods, or techniques for physical or psychological development. His teachings do not provide solutions to material, economic, psychological, emotional, familial, social, or bodily problems. Prabhuji does not promise miracles or spiritual salvation. He only talks about what happened to him and shares his own experience fraternally through his books and video conferences.

A group of senior disciples and friends voluntarily contribute to preserve Prabhuji's vision, message, and legacy for future generations. According to their humble possibilities, they cooperate in the distribution of his books, websites, and videos of talks given to small groups of disciples in the Prabhuji Ashram.

We ask everyone to respect his privacy and not to try to contact him, by any means, for interviews, blessings, *śaktipāta*, initiations, or personal visits.

Titles by Prabhuji

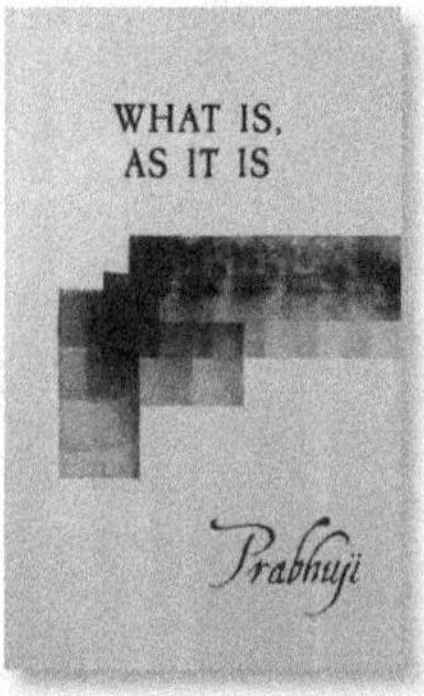

What is, as it is: Satsangs with Prabhuji (English)
ISBN-13:978-0-9815264-4-7
Lo que es, tal como es: Satsangs con Prabhuji (Spanish)
ISBN-13:978-0-9815264-5-4
Russian: ISBN-13: 978-1-945894-18-3

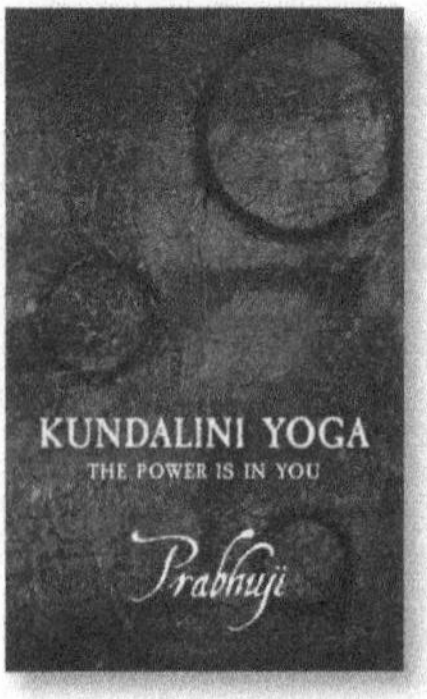

Kundalini yoga: The power is in you (English)
ISBN-13:978-1-945894-02-2
Kundalini yoga: El poder está en ti (Spanish)
ISBN-13:978-1-945894-01-5

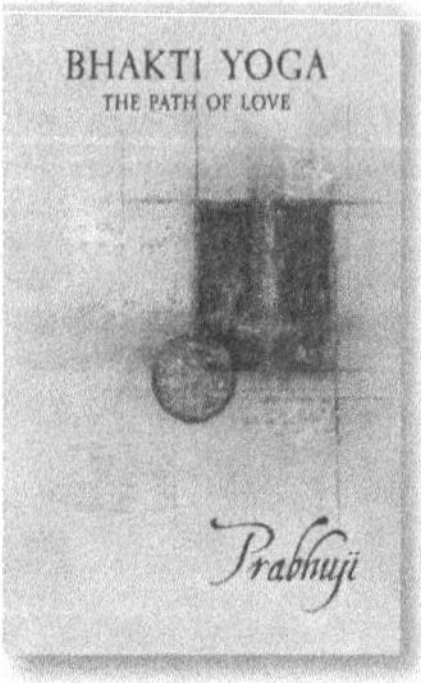

Bhakti yoga: The path of love (English)
ISBN-13:978-1-945894-03-9
Bhakti-yoga: El sendero del amor (Spanish)
ISBN-13:978-1-945894-04-6

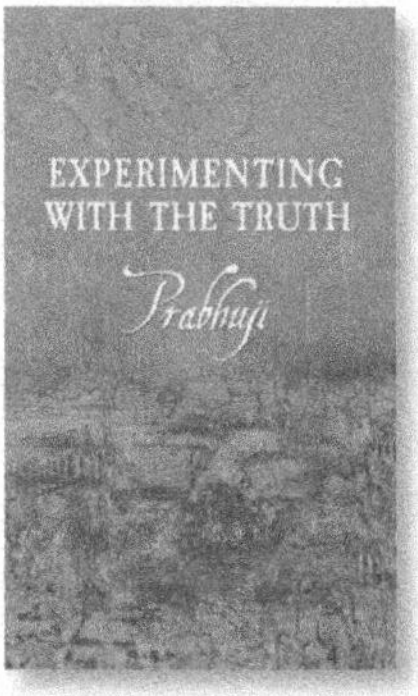

Experimenting with the Truth (English)
ISBN-13: 978-1-945894-08-4
Experimentando con la Verdad (Spanish)
ISBN-13: 978-1-945894-09-1

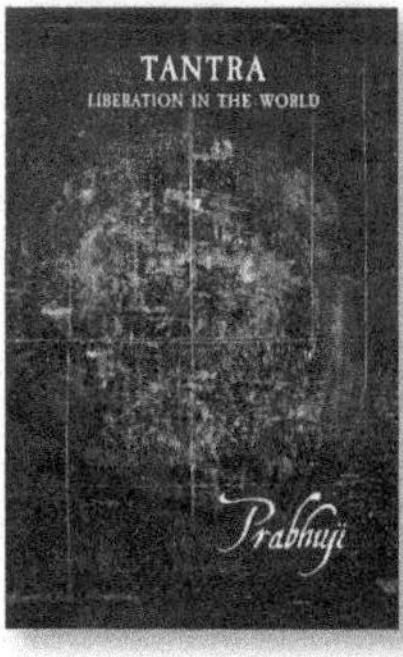

Tantra: Liberation in the world (English)
ISBN-13: 978-1-945894-21-3
Tantra: La liberación en el mundo (Spanish)
ISBN-13: 978-1-945894-23-7

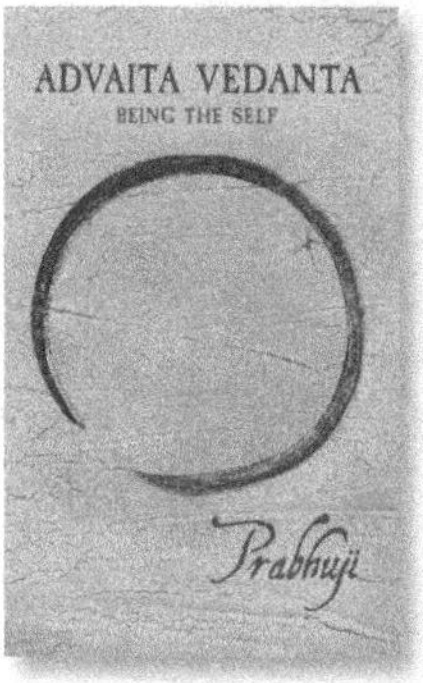

Advaita Vedanta: Being the Self (English)
ISBN-13: 978-1-945894-20-6
Advaita Vedanta: Ser el Ser (Spanish)
ISBN-13: 978-1-945894-16-9

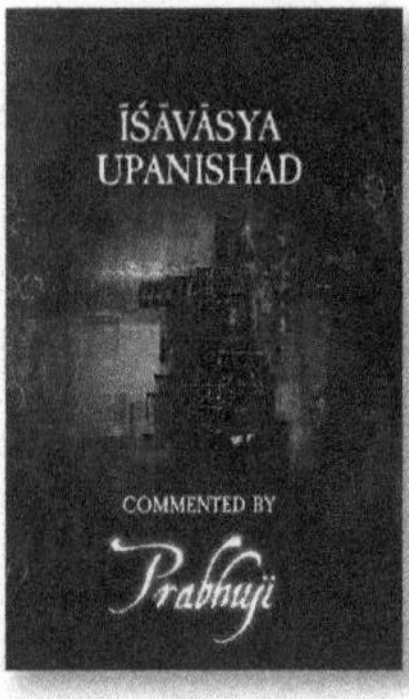

Īśāvāsya Upanishad
commented by Prabhuji
(English)
ISBN-13: 978-1-945894-39-8
Īśāvāsya Upaniṣad
comentado by Prabhuji
(Spanish)
ISBN-13: 978-1-945894-41-1

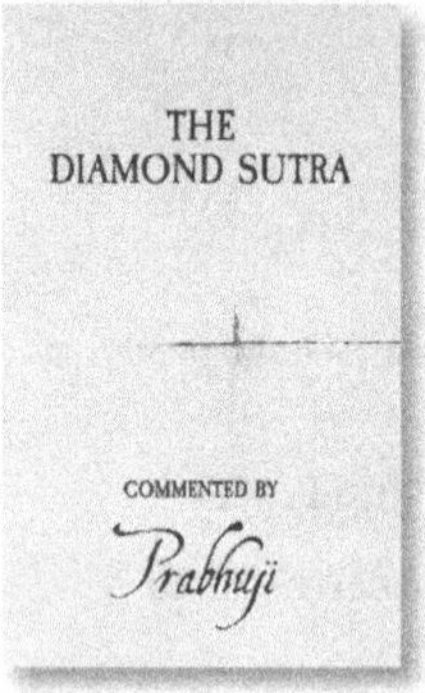

Diamond Sutra
Commented by Prabhuji
Coming soon!